Managing Acute Mania

RK Morriss (Editor)
University of Liverpool, Liverpool, UK

JC Cookson
Royal London Hospital, London UK

IN Ferrier, K Macritchie, AH Young
University of Newcastle-upon-Tyne, Newcastle-upon-Tyne, UK

ML Phillips, MJ Travis
Institute of Psychiatry, London, UK

SP
SCIENCE
PRESS

Published by Science Press Ltd, 34–42 Cleveland Street, London W1T 4LB, UK.

© 2003 Science Press Ltd

http://www.science-press.com/

British Library Cataloguing in Publication Data.

A catalogue record for this book is available from the British Library.

ISBN 1-85873-991-8

Although every effort has been made to ensure that drug doses and other information are presented accurately in this publication, the ultimate responsibility rests with the prescribing physician. Neither the publishers nor the authors can be held responsible for errors or for any consequences arising from the use of information contained herein. Any product mentioned in this publication should be used in accordance with the prescribing information prepared by the manufacturers. No claims or endorsements are made for any drug or compound at present under clinical investigation.

Project editor: Clare Wheatcroft
Project co-ordinator: Ronit Shafron
Illustrator: Matthew McCutcheon
Designer: Simon Banister
Production: Adrienne Hanratty

Printed in the UK by Halstan & Co.

Cover illustration: Abstract image with horizontal lines. © Royalty-Free/CORBIS.

Contents

Author biographies

Editor

Professor Richard K Morriss is Professor of Psychiatry and Head of Department at the University of Liverpool, Liverpool, UK. He qualified in medicine from the University of Leeds, Leeds, UK. He trained in psychiatry in Leeds, Oxford and Manchester, UK, where he was a lecturer. He also held a research fellowship in neuropsychiatry at Johns Hopkins University, Baltimore, Maryland, USA. He was appointed a senior lecturer at the University of Manchester, Manchester, UK with consultant psychiatrist duties in Preston, Lancashire, UK, before being appointed to his Chair in 1999. Professor Morriss has developed research and clinical interests in the management of bipolar affective disorder, somatization, chronic fatigue syndrome and primary care psychiatry, including studies of the outcome of psychosocial interventions and the training of health professionals in the management of these disorders.

Contributors

Dr John C Cookson is Consultant in General Adult Psychiatry at the Royal London Hospital, in East London, UK, where he has worked since 1981. He won the Theodore Williams Scholarship in physiology at Oxford University. After completing a doctorate in the pharmacology of neuromuscular transmission at Oxford, he studied clinical medicine at University College Hospital, London, UK. He continued higher training at St Bartholomew's and the Maudsley Hospitals, London, UK. Dr Cookson is responsible for a catchment area service, comprising a community mental health team and a general psychiatric ward, and for a Psychiatric Intensive Care Unit. He also has responsibility in the Drug Dependency service. He has co-authored the fifth edition of *The Use of Drugs in Psychiatry: Evidence from Psychopharmacology*, published by the Royal College of Psychiatrists, 2002. His main research interests are in psychopharmacology and the use of drugs in psychiatry, particularly in relation to the treatment of bipolar affective disorder. He has also participated in the development of new drugs for schizophrenia and panic disorder, and in studies of neuroendocrinology. He has served on the editorial boards of the *British Journal of Psychiatry*, *International Clinical Psychopharmacology* and *Advances in Psychiatric Treatment*.

Professor I Nicol Ferrier studied physiology and medicine at the University of Glasgow, Glasgow, UK. After training in general medicine in Glasgow he moved to London and trained in psychiatry under the supervision of Professors Tim Crow and Eve Johnstone. He held Medical Research Council (MRC) and Wellcome Training Fellowships carrying out research on the neurochemistry and neuroendocrinology of schizophrenia. In 1983, he was awarded his MD with honours from the University of Glasgow. In 1984, he moved to Newcastle as an MRC Clinical Scientist to the then MRC Neuroendocrinology Unit, Newcastle, UK. In 1990, he was appointed as Professor of Psychiatry at the University of Newcastle-upon-Tyne and became Head of Department in 1996. In 2002, he was appointed as Head of the School of Neurology, Neurobiology and Psychiatry. He was appointed as a Fellow of the Royal College of Psychiatrists in 1990 and a Fellow of the Royal College of Physicians of Edinburgh in 1996. Professor Ferrier is Director of the Stanley Bipolar Research Centre in Newcastle, UK. He is the General Secretary of the British Association for Psychopharmacology and a member of the MRC Training Awards Panel, National Institute of Clinical Excellence (NICE) Guidelines for Depression Committee and was a member of the Psychiatry subpanel of the Research Assessment Exercise 2001. His interests include the neurobiology and treatment of severe affective disorders.

Dr Karine Macritchie studied physiology and medicine at the University of Glasgow, Glasgow, UK. After training in general practice she undertook basic training in psychiatry in Cambridge, UK. There, she completed a six-month research post investigating the existence of anticonvulsant 'rebound' mania and established an interest in evidence-based medicine examining the efficacy of mood stabilizers in bipolar affective disorder through the Cochrane Reviews. She joined the Northern Region Specialist Training Scheme in 2000. Subsequently, she worked in the Chronic Affective Disorders Unit at the Royal Victoria Infirmary, Newcastle-upon-Tyne, UK. Currently, she is a Clinical Research Associate in the Stanley Bipolar Research Centre at the University of Newcastle-upon-Tyne, Newcastle, UK, where she is engaged on a neuroimaging project in bipolar patients.

Dr Mary L Phillips is Director of a bipolar service for North East Lambeth, London, UK at the Maudsley Hospital, London, UK and Senior Lecturer and Honorary Consultant in the Division of Psychological Medicine, Institute of Psychiatry (IOP) and Guy's, King's and St Thomas' School of Medicine, London, UK. Dr Phillips trained in medicine at Cambridge and in psychiatry at the Royal Bethlem and Maudsley Hospitals. Her research interests from 1996 have been the investigation of facial perception using functional magnetic resonance imaging (fMRI) and from 1997 the investigation of emotion perception using fMRI. Since 1998 Dr Phillips and her group have initiated a programme of research funded by the Wellcome Trust, The Pilkington Foundation and Unilever, amongst others, investigating the neural correlates of abnormal emotion perception in different psychiatric populations with fMRI. The groups include patients suffering from bipolar disorder, schizophrenia, phobias, obsessive compulsive disorder and depersonalization disorder. She is involved in a number of national and international collaborative research projects.

Dr Mike J Travis is a lecturer in clinical neuropharmacology and consultant psychiatrist at London's Institute of Psychiatry and Maudsley Hospital, London, UK. Dr Travis trained in medicine at Guy's Hospital and in psychiatry at St Bartholomew's and Hackney Hospitals and the Royal Bethlem and Maudsley Hospitals, London, UK. In his research activities his main interest is the study of drug action using functional imaging. His most recent contributions have been in the development of a novel ligand for the serotonin-2A receptor for single photon emission tomography (SPET) and its use in clinical populations. His clinical interests are in clinical psychopharmacology and psychiatric intensive care. He has published several book chapters in addition to original experimental research. He is currently involved in studies analysing the relationship between dopamine-D-2 receptor availability and treatment response in schizophrenia, in addition to studies investigating the neurochemical basis of Asperger's syndrome and the effects of hormone replacement therapy on cortical serotonin-2A receptors and muscarinic receptors.

Professor Allan H Young trained in medicine and thereafter psychiatry at the University of Edinburgh and held a Royal College of Physicians of Edinburgh training fellowship at the MRC Brain Metabolism Unit, Edinburgh, UK. Subsequently, he was a clinical lecturer at the University of Oxford, Oxford, UK and worked in the MRC Clinical Psychopharmacology Unit with Professor Philip Cowen before becoming senior lecturer and honorary consultant at the University of Newcastle-upon-Tyne, Newcastle, UK. Now Professor of General Psychiatry, Allan Young is also Director of the Stanley Bipolar Research Centre in Newcastle, Newcastle, UK. He is a Council Member of the British Association for Psychopharmacology, Secretary of the Royal College of Psychiatrists' Psychopharmacology Special Interest Group and member of the Scientific Advisory Council of the Stanley Medical Research Institute. He has published over 200 scientific publications on the aetiology and treatment of psychiatric disorders, particularly mood disorders.

Chapter 1

Introduction to acute mania

IN Ferrier

A brief history of the term 'mania'

The origin of the concept of bipolar disorder has its roots in the views of Greek physicians of the classical period. Mania is one of the earliest described human diseases. The description of Aretaeus of Cappadocia (circa AD90) captures both the core and the range of key symptoms:

> *'Some patients with mania are cheerful, they laugh, play, dance day and night, they stroll in the market, sometimes with a garland on the head, as if they had been winner in a game: these patients do not bring worries to their relatives. But others fly into rage... The manifestations of mania are countless. Some manics, who are intelligent and well educated, are dealing with astronomy, although they never studied it...'*

The origins of the term 'mania' are unclear and from the outset until the present day the term has been used in a broad way. The classical physicians used the term 'mania' with different meanings, such as a reaction to an event (eg, rage, anger), a biologically defined disease (Hippocrates felt mania was a disease of the brain), a divine state and, especially in its mild form, a temperament [1].

In the early 1900s Kraepelin developed the concept of manic-depressive insanity characterized by the course and prognosis of the disease. For Kraepelin a good prognosis was essential to the definition of manic-depressive illness, although recent research has questioned this as poor psychosocial function and persistent symptoms have been found in many patients. Kraepelin was convinced that symptoms were of little value for the diagnosis and highlighted the particular problem of the range of psychiatric symptoms in mania. He described mania as an acceleration of three functions (mood regulation, cognition and psychomotor activity) and opined that mixed states were due to asynchronous oscillations in each of these functions.

In 1957, Leonhard proposed a clinical classification that went beyond clinical description alone and he coined the term 'bipolar' for those patients with a history of mania. In 1966 Angst [2] and Perris [3] independently demonstrated that unipolar disorder and bipolar disorder could be differentiated in terms of clinical presentation, evolution, family history and therapeutic response. This led through a series of steps, to the categorization of bipolar disorder in *Diagnostic and Statistical Manual of Mental Disorders* (DSM), now in its fourth edition (DSM-IV) [4] and to the broadening of the concept to describe and delineate clinical syndromes, such as schizo-affective psychoses, mixed states and the bipolar spectrum disorders. A further expansion has led to the categories of bipolar I disorder (at least one manic episode) and bipolar II disorder (at least one hypomanic episode).

Clinical features of mania

Mania is a complex disorder with many facets to its clinical presentation. The diagnostic criteria for a manic episode are shown in Table 1.1. DSM-IV specifically states that manic episodes which are clearly precipitated by antidepressant treatment (eg, pharmacotherapy, electroconvulsive therapy [ECT]) are not indicative of bipolar I disorder. Many have suggested, however, that such episodes should be treated in the short and longer term as if they were part of a bipolar I condition. The range of symptoms in mania has been well described by Goodwin and Jamison [5] and their findings are summarized in Table 1.2. The severity of mania is such that there is marked impairment in occupational functioning.

Criteria for manic episode	
Category	**Description**
A	A distinct period of abnormally and persistently elevated, expansive or irritable mood, lasting at least one week (or any duration if hospitalization is necessary)
B	During the period of mood disturbance, three (or more) of the following symptoms have persisted (four if the mood is only irritable) and have been present to a significant degree 1. inflated self-esteem or grandiosity 2. decreased need for sleep (eg, feels rested after only three hours of sleep) 3. more talkative than usual or pressure to keep talking 4. flight of ideas or subjective experience that thoughts are racing 5. distractibility (ie, attention too easily drawn to unimportant or irrelevant external stimuli) 6. increase in goal-directed activity (either socially, at work or school, or sexually) or psychomotor agitation 7. excessive involvement in pleasurable activities that have a high potential for painful consequences (eg, engaging in unrestrained buying sprees, sexual indiscretions or foolish business investments)
C	The symptoms do not meet criteria for a mixed episode
D	The mood disturbance is sufficiently severe to cause marked impairment in occupational functioning or in usual social activities or relationships with others or to necessitate hospitalization to prevent harm to self or others or there are psychotic features
E	The symptoms are not due to the direct physiological effects of a substance (eg, a drug abuse, a medication or other treatment) or a general medical condition (eg, hyperthyroidism)

Table 1.1. Note that manic-like episodes that are clearly caused by somatic antidepressant treatment (eg, medication, electroconvulsive therapy, light therapy) should not count toward a diagnosis of bipolar I disorder. Reproduced with permission from *Diagnostic and Statistical Manual of Mental Disorders. Fourth edition.* Washington, DC: American Psychiatric Association; 1994 [4].

Manic episodes: mean rate of symptom occurrence			
Mood symptoms:		**History of psychotic symptoms**	58%
Irritability	80%	**Thought disorder**	19%
Euphoria	71%	**First rank symptoms (Schneider)**	18%
Depression	72%	**Activity and behaviour during mania:**	
Lability	69%	Hyperactivity	87%
Expansiveness	60%	Decreased sleep	81%
Cognitive symptoms:		Violent assaultive behaviour	49%
Grandiosity	78%	Rapid pressured speech	98%
Flight of ideas, racing thoughts	71%	Hyperverbosity	89%
Distractibility, poor concentration	71%	Nudity, sexual exposure	29%
Confusion	25%	Hypersexuality	57%
Psychotic symptoms:		Extravagance	55%
Any delusion	48%	Religiosity	39%
Grandiosity	47%	Head decoration	34%
Persecutory paranoid	28%	Regression (pronounced)	28%
Passivity	15%	Catatonia	22%
Any hallucinations	15%	Faecal incontinence (smearing)	13%
Auditory hallucinations	18%		
Visual hallucinations	10%		
Olfactory hallucinations	17%		

Table 1.2. Adapted with permission from Goodwin FK, Jamison KR. *Manic-depressive Illness.* New York: Oxford University Press; 1990 [5].

Various subtypes of mania are said to exist, but their boundaries have not been formally validated. These include:

- euphoric (classic) mania;
- irritable mania;
- dysphoric mania; and
- mixed states.

There may be prognostic and therapeutic implications to these distinctions some of which are discussed in this book. Most authorities distinguish mania with and without psychotic features. It is important to recognise that mood incongruent psychotic features (including Schneiderian first-rank symptoms) can occur in mania. Psychosis in mania occurs in approximately 70% of cases on a lifetime basis and in approximately 50% of cases at any one time-point. Psychosis acts as a course-modifier and is associated with an increased relapse rate [6], but it is not clear if its presence alters treatment choices and many would argue that it does not. If a patient is severely manic and psychotic, however, the case for antipsychotic therapy would be strong. Another type of mania that has been described is mania with and without catatonia, but the validity of this distinction and its prognostic and therapeutic implications have not been established.

It is important to recognise that bipolar disorder is often comorbid with other disorders, such as substance abuse and anxiety, and, therefore, the clinical picture of mania may be 'contaminated' by the presence of these additional disorders.

In bipolar disorder, approximately 50% of first episodes are manic and the median age of onset is in the late teens. Between 10% and 20% of patients classified as having recurrent depressive disorder have a subsequent manic episode. In this population, the mean number of episodes before 'switching' is three [3]. The switch can occur at any age, but occurs in the majority of patients by their early thirties [5].

Episodes of mania can last for between four and 13 months; the longer periods are from studies before drug treatments were available. Most studies suggest that manic episodes are shorter than depressive episodes and that manic episodes become shorter as the patient gets older. Episodes can be very severe leading to exhaustion and, rarely, death and, although now infrequent, chronic mania can occur.

Hypomania

Hypomania is an attenuated form of mania and, by definition, is not associated with psychosis. The DSM-IV criteria for hypomania are given in Table 1.3. The key distinctions between mania and hypomania are that hypomania can be diagnosed after four days and that, while the disorder is associated with an unequivocal change in functioning, there is no marked impairment. Consequently, hypomania is often undiagnosed. Goodwin [7] has elegantly argued that the boundaries 'above' and 'below' hypomania are uncertain; this is a matter of great importance as there are associated treatment issues. For example, it is not clear at what degree hypomanic symptoms necessitate treatment. The absence of a good marker of severity combined with a problematic evidence base also leads to uncertainty and inappropriate prescribing, which occurs at an unknown frequency. Similarly it is not clear which level of hypomania should lead to cautions on the use of antidepressants developed for mania, marked hypomania or mixed states (ie, in patients with recurrent depression and mild hypomania at what point should mood stabilizers rather than long-term antidepressant drugs be advised). It is important to recognise that the vast majority of treatment studies involve mania; when and how to extend this evidence base into hypomania is a matter for clinical judgement. The presence of hypomania also impacts on the use of antidepressant

	DSM-IV criteria for hypomania
Category	**Description**
A	A distinct period of persistently elevated, expansive or irritable mood, lasting throughout at least four days that is clearly different from the usual nondepressed mood
B	During the period of mood disturbance, three (or more) of the following symptoms have persisted (four if the mood is only irritable) and have been present to a significant degree: 1. inflated self-esteem or grandiosity 2. decreased need for sleep (eg, feels rested after only three hours of sleep) 3. more talkative than usual or pressure to keep talking 4. flight of ideas or subjective experience that thoughts are racing 5. distractibility (ie, attention too easily drawn to unimportant or irrelevant external stimuli) 6. increase goal-directed activity (either socially, at work or school, or sexually) or psychomotor agitation 7. excessive involvement in pleasurable activities that have a high potential for painful consequences (eg, the person engages in unrestrained buying sprees, sexual indiscretion or foolish business investment)
C	The episode is associated with an unequivocal change in functioning that is uncharacteristic of the person when not symptomatic
D	The disturbance in mood and the change in functioning are observable by others
E	The episode is not severe enough to cause marked impairment in social or occupational functioning or to necessitate hospitalization and there are no psychotic features
F	The symptoms are not due to the direct physiological effects of a substance (eg, a drug abuse, a medication or other treatment) or a general medical condition (eg, hyperthyroidism)

Table 1.3. Note that hypomanic-like episodes that are clearly caused by somatic anti-depressant treatment (eg, medication, electroconvulsive therapy, light therapy) should not count toward a diagnosis of bipolar II disorder. Reproduced with permission from American Psychiatric Association. *Diagnostic and Statistical Manual of Mental Disorders. Fourth edition. (DSM-IV)* Washington, DC: American Psychiatric Association; 1994 [4].

agents as these may speed up cycling in bipolar II disorder. Rapid-cycling disorder is defined by the occurrence of four or more affective episodes in 12 months. Rapid-cycling disorder is thought to occur in up to 25% of bipolar patients and may be becoming more common.

Secondary mania

Krauthammer and Klerman [8] coined the term 'secondary mania' to classify manic symptoms closely associated temporally with systemic medical or neurological conditions. The DSM-IV [4] translates this concept into the category of 'mood disorder due to a medical condition' with the presumption that the disturbance is the direct physiological consequence of a general medical condition. Factors that are associated with this are a negative family history, no prior history of mood disorder and a late age of onset. A specific physical condition occurring in a patient with affective vulnerability may be the relevant mechanism in the majority of patients, which may explain the relative rarity of this condition. The prognosis is variable, but cognitive impairment is commonplace and there is suggestion that the response to treatment is less good than in primary mania. Secondary mania is often associated with underlying cardiovascular pathology in elderly patients. Secondary mania is associated with cerebral infarctions and with subcortical white matter hyperintensities (although it is noteworthy that the latter also occur in young-onset bipolar patients with no evidence of underlying vascular disease). In some patients, secondary mania has been described as 'vascular' mania. There is evidence that vascular lesions on the right side of the brain in vulnerable individuals may produce a syndrome of disinhibition and pathological laughing.

The nature and type of medical conditions associated with secondary mania is heterogeneous. Currently only small case series and individual case reports have been published. A list of drugs that have been implicated in secondary mania is shown in Table 1.4 [9]. Comorbidity rates with substance abuse are high and can create diagnostic problems, but in many cases, the underlying bipolar disorder is the main issue. Alcohol abuse is associated with a poor prognosis, but the mechanism for the poor outcome is probably multifactorial, including poor compliance as well as the impact of alcohol excess and withdrawal on mental state, cognition and drug efficacy. There is, however, evidence that appropriate treatment of the substance abuse improves bipolar outcome and compliance [10].

Drugs associated with manic symptoms	
Amphetamines	Hallucinogens (intoxication and flashbacks)
Baclofen	Hydralazine
Bromide	Isoniazid
Bromocriptine	Levodopa
Captopril	Methylphenidate
Cimetidine	Metrizamide (following myelography)
Cocaine	Opiates and opioids
Corticosteroids (including ACTH)	Procarbazine
Ciclosporin	Procyclidine
Disulfiram	

Table 1.4. ACTH, adrenocorticotrophic hormone. Reproduced with permission from Kaplan HI, Sadock BJ, Grebb JA. *Kaplan and Sadock's Synopsis of Psychiatry. Behavioral Sciences Clinical Psychiatry. Seventh edition.* Baltimore: Williams & Wilkins; 1994 [9].

The medical conditions and lesions associated with secondary mania are listed in Table 1.5. Cases in which the suspicion of a secondary mania is raised should be investigated. Treatment is primarily symptomatic, but has similarities with the management of primary cases outlined in subsequent chapters of this book.

Organic (secondary) causes of manic and hypomanic symptoms	
Metabolic disturbance	**Neoplasm**
Postoperative states	Parasagittal meningioma
Haemodialysis	Diencephalic glioma
Vitamin B12 deficiency	Suprasellar craniopharyngioma
Addison's disease	Suprasellar diencephalic tumour
Cushing's disease	Benign spheno-occipital tumour
Postinfection states	Right intraventricular meningioma
Dialysis	Right temporoparietal occipital metastases
Hyperthyroidism	Tumour of floor of fourth ventricle
Neurological conditions	**Other conditions**
Right-temporal seizure focus	Postisolation syndrome
Multiple sclerosis	Right temporal lobectomy
Right-hemisphere damage	Post-traumatic confusion
Epilepsy	Post-electroconvulsive therapy
Huntingdon's disease	Deliriform organic brain disease
Postcerebrovascular accident	
Infection	
Influenza	
Q fever	
Neurosyphilis	
Post-St Louis type A encephalitis	
'Benign' herpes simplex encephalitis	
AIDS (HIV)	

Table 1.5. AIDS, acquired immunodeficiency syndrome; HIV, human immunodeficiency virus. Adapted with permission from Goodwin FK, Jamison KR. *Manic-depressive Illness.* New York: Oxford University Press; 1990 [5].

References

1. Angst J, Marneros A. **Bipolarity from ancient to modern times: conception, birth and rebirth.** *J Affect Disord* 2001; **67**:3–19.

2. Angst J. *Zur Atiologie und Nosologie Endogener Depressiver Psychosen.* Berlin: Springer; 1966.

3. Perris C. **A study of bipolar (manic-depressive) and unipolar recurrent depressive psychoses. Introduction.** *Acta Psychiatr Scand Suppl* 1966; **194**:9–14.

4. American Psychiatric Association. *Diagnostic and Statistical Manual of Mental Disorders. Fourth edition (DSM-IV).* Washington, DC: American Psychiatric Association; 1994.

5. Goodwin FK, Jamison KR. *Manic-depressive Illness.* New York: Oxford University Press; 1990.

6. Tohen M, Waternaux CM, Tsuang MT. **Outcome in mania. A 4-year prospective follow-up of 75 patients utilizing survival analysis.** *Arch Gen Psychiatry* 1990; **47**:1106–1111.

7. Goodwin G. **Hypomania: what's in a name.** *Br J Psychiatry* 2002; **181**:94–95.

8. Krauthammer C, Klerman GL. **Secondary mania: manic syndromes associated with antecedent physical illness or drugs.** *Arch Gen Psychiatry* 1978; **35**:1333–1339.

9. Kaplan HI, Sadock BJ, Grebb JA. *Kaplan and Sadock's Synopsis of Psychiatry. Behavioral Sciences Clinical Psychiatry. Seventh edition.* Baltimore: Williams & Wilkins; 1994.

10. Liskow B, Mayfield D, Thiele J. **Alcohol and affective disorder: assessment and treatment.** *J Clin Psychiatry* 1982; **43**:144–147.

Chapter 2

Problems of initial management

RK Morriss

Importance of obtaining previous history

The diagnosis of mania can be muddled with other disorders, such as those shown in Table 2.1. A longitudinal history can clarify the diagnosis. For example, a previous history of depressive episodes or mania can help to clarify the current diagnosis of mania as opposed to a drug-induced psychosis when there has been concomitant use of illicit stimulants or antidepressant agents.

Differential diagnosis of mania
Schizophrenia or other non-affective psychosis
Drug- or alcohol-induced psychosis
Drug- or alcohol-induced mania
Drug or alcohol intoxication
Drug or alcohol withdrawal
Medical disorder-induced mania (eg, stroke, multiple sclerosis)
Iatrogenic-induced mania (eg, prescribed steroids, antidepressant agents)
Delirium (acute confusional state; eg, after head injury, infection)
Puerperal psychosis

Table 2.1

A recent longitudinal history can indicate the best treatment approach and likely prognosis. A current manic episode may be preceded by a well phase or a depressed phase. It can also be considered as a phase of a rapid-cycling bipolar affective disorder (four or more mood episodes per year). Mania may be induced by antidepressant or stimulant drugs (prescribed or over the counter, for example, St John's Wort or illicit drugs). If this is the case then these drugs should be stopped as part of the clinical management [1]. A history of a preceding depressive episode would suggest the use of a mood stabilizer rather than a typical antipsychotic drug to prevent switching from mania immediately into a depressed episode [2]. When mania is a phase of a rapid-cycling mood state or there is a recent history of many previous episodes, an anticonvulsant drug known to be effective against rapid cycling, such as valproate or carbamazepine, should be used rather than lithium or antipsychotic drugs [3]. Previous treatment response to the variety of anti-manic agents that are now available may be a guide to other agents that are likely to be effective in the current episode for a particular patient. In terms of prognosis, a history of prominent dysphoric symptoms or psychotic features may suggest a more prolonged course for the current episode of mania [4–6].

Previous history can be obtained from the patient, but the patient's mental state may preclude the taking of a clear history because they may be too restless, agitated, disinhibited, grandiose, deluded or incoherent. Other sources of previous history are shown in Table 2.2.

Sources of previous history
Carer
Relative or friend
Key worker (mental health professional who follows up patient)
General practitioner
Psychiatry case notes
General practitioner notes
Written or computerized care plans (care programme approach after multidisciplinary case conference, a copy of which may be available on a networked computer or patient and carer may hold copies)

Table 2.2

Among the most important reasons for obtaining previous history are the assessment of risk to the patient or other people, including staff members. Risks to the patient in the current episode of mania are probably similar to the risks in previous episodes of mania. The nature of these risks is shown in Table 2.3. These should be confirmed by:

- mental state examination (eg, suicide risk, risk to others);

- physical examination (eg, clinical signs of dehydration, poor nutritional state); and

- relevant investigations (eg, urea and electrolytes for dehydration, random blood glucose for poor diabetic control, hepatitis B or C status).

A previous history may reveal the existence of an advanced directive concerning how the patient should be treated if they become ill. The directive should be signed in the presence of the patient's consultant psychiatrist and witnessed by another person to demonstrate they were well and able to make such decisions. An advanced directive should be followed, unless it would put the patient or others, including staff and other patients, at risk of their health, wellbeing or safety.

Risks to patient and others from mania
Risks to patient
Suicide (brief periods of depression and irritability are common in mania)
Through misjudgement/recklessness (eg, driving over speed limit and ignoring traffic lights and signs), becoming pregnant or contracting a sexually transmitted disease through sexual indiscretion
Other people reacting aggressively to the disinhibited behaviour of the patient with mania
Self-neglect, dehydration and poor nutritional state
Self-neglect, disinhibition and overactivity in medically unwell patient (eg, patient with diabetes neglects dietary control)
Overspending or irresponsible spending of personal finances
Risks to others
Irritability is common in mania and can lead to aggression and violence (particularly in people who already have a low threshold for violence)
Recklessness, misjudgement and disinhibition leading to:
• Abandonment, neglect or mistreatment of dependent vulnerable people usually cared for by the patient (eg, babies and children, disabled and elderly)
• Neglect or mistreatment of others at work
• Overspending or irresponsible spending of family or work finances
• Reckless behaviour in people who pose medical risks to other people (eg, sexual indiscretion in people who are positive for human immunodeficiency virus or hepatitis B or C infection)

Table 2.3

Patients with bipolar disorder may have other comorbid psychiatric or medical problems, detailed in Table 2.4. It is important for the immediate management of the patient with mania that these conditions are known about. Knowledge of these may be obtained from a previous history.

Finally, a previous history can sometimes identify important psychosocial factors leading to manic relapse:

1. life stressors that disrupt circadian rhythms (eg, shift work or flying across time zones);

2. family or life stressors that direct hostility and criticism to the patient; and

3. good and poor coping mechanisms with the early or prodromal symptoms of mania that are known to decrease or increase the need for admission because of mania [7].

These are important in the immediate management of the patient with mania if the stressors are ongoing (eg, life stress at home may mean that home treatment is

Psychiatric and medical comorbidity complicating treatment of mania	
Type of comorbidity	**Complication**
Alcohol or drug misuse	Increased risk of suicide and violence, poor adherence to treatment
Anxiety disorders	Increased side effects from medication
Personality disorder	Increased risk of suicide and violence, poor adherence to treatment
Neuroleptic malignant syndrome (rigidity, stupor, high temperature rise, autonomic instability)	Caution in use of antipsychotic drugs and lithium
Tardive dyskinesia	Caution in use of antipsychotic drugs
Renal impairment and/or inappropriate antidiuretic hormone release	Caution in use of lithium
Thyroid disease	Caution in use of lithium
Cardiac disease	Caution in use of lithium, carbamazepine and antipsychotic drugs
Addison's disease	Caution in use of lithium
Myasthenia gravis	Caution in use of lithium
Diabetes mellitus/obesity	Caution in use of olanzapine, lithium and valproate
Hepatic impairment	Caution in use of valproate
Haematological disorder	Caution in use of valproate and carbamazepine

Table 2.4

inadvisable). It is also important that they are recognised in after care to prevent further episodes of mania [8].

Procedures to keep patients with mania under control

Voluntary (medical) admission

Home treatment is not a suitable alternative to hospital admission for patients with mania who are highly active, disinhibited, reckless or requiring little sleep. The amount of sedation required to reduce overactivity should be continuously supervised by nursing staff with medical support. Mania is usually a highly unpredictable mental state that exhausts carers who require more rest and sleep than the patient. The patient needs to be constantly engaged in activity with a low threshold for harm and in a non-stimulating environment providing few distractions. Such conditions are rarely available at home or in respite care, so the patient is almost invariably admitted to hospital. An exception is the patient with mania who has psychotic features and is not disinhibited, reckless or overactive. Such patients may on occasion be managed at home by carers who are willing and able to sustain support and supervision throughout most of the day for a number of weeks. The carers require the input of home treatment teams containing nursing and medical staff, a member of which is able to visit the home at least twice per day.

Voluntary admission is possible when the patient retains sufficient insight to recognise that they are in a manic state (ie, this state is abnormal) and to give informed consent to staying in hospital, taking medication and restriction in the nature and level of activities. Consent to voluntary admission can be inferred in patients who make no attempt to leave the in-patient unit, do not engage in activities that may directly lead to harm to themselves or others and accept treatment, including medication, without protest [9]. Repeated reckless behaviour likely to compromise the safety of the patient or other people or refusal of treatment, including medication, will require an assessment and probably detention of the patient under the Mental Health Act law. An isolated incident of reckless behaviour without serious consequences may be managed under common law without assessment under the Mental Health Act law.

Involuntary (legal) admission

At present, the Mental Health Act law in England and Wales is under review. Although the details of the process by which a patient with mania is detained may change when a new mental health act is passed, the conditions under which it is appropriate to detain a patient with mania in hospital against their will are unlikely to differ substantially from the current guidelines. The criteria by which a patient with mania can be currently detained, and the legal processes involved, are shown in Table 2.5. There are separate provisions for criminal law cases.

Treatment for mania, covered by the 1983 Mental Health Act in England and Wales [10], includes both acute and continuation psychotropic medication delivered orally or parenterally for up to three months, but electroconvulsive therapy (ECT) requires additional use of the 1983 Mental Health Act. Treatment also includes containment on the ward, if necessary under more secure conditions, to prevent reckless, aggressive or self-injurious behaviour.

By definition, treatment of mania on a locked ward requires the patient to be detained under the 1983 Mental Health Act. Under some instances in other countries voluntary patients can be admitted to locked wards. Where the facilities are available, transfer of the detained patient to a more secure ward ('psychiatric intensive care') can be beneficial. There is improved security, a higher staff-to-patient ratio providing opportunities to contain behaviour and properly monitor medication, and quieter wards with less stimulation and fewer distractions.

Use of 1983 Mental Health Act in England and Wales for mania			
Legislation	**Criteria**	**Application**	**Effect**
Admission for assessment, section 2	Mental disorder warrants detention in hospital for assessment + risk to health or safety of patient or others	Approved social worker or nearest relative + medical recommendations from two doctors, one is section 12 approved	Patient detained for 28 days for assessment and treatment can be started
Admission for treatment, section 3	Mental illness of nature and severity that makes medical treatment in hospital appropriate (usually defined on similar lines to section 2)	Approved social worker (but not if nearest relative objects) + two medical recommendations, one from section 12 approved doctor	Patient detained for six months, but detention renewable
Admission for assessment in emergency, section 4	Urgent admission for assessment (should be rarely required)	Approved social worker or nearest relative + one recommendation (preferably from doctor who knows patient)	72 hours unless second medical opinion received (then 28 days, but treatment cannot be started)
Patients already in hospital, section 5.2	Patient already voluntarily admitted to hospital (not casualty) who requires compulsory detention because of risk	RMO or nominated deputy	72 hours. Treatment cannot be started
Nurses holding power, section 5.4	Patient already voluntarily admitted to hospital, at risk to self or others if allowed to leave, impractical to obtain RMO or nominated deputy immediately	Qualified nurse with training and experience in mental health	Six hours or until arrival of doctor. Treatment cannot be started
Treatment requiring consent or second opinion, section 58	Patients under section 3 who may receive ECT or medication after three months of treatment	RMO or independent doctor certifies that patient has given and is capable of providing written informed consent or independent doctor agrees treatment should be given to alleviate or prevent deterioration	Course of ECT or medication given for longer than three months

Table 2.5. RMO, responsible medical officer; ECT, electroconvulsive therapy.

Shared care, co-ordination and communication

Relatives

Relatives are usually an important source of information about the patient. There are, however, issues of confidentiality that need to be considered before any discussion of a patient occurs with a relative. In British mental health practice, a carer who lives with the patient or has a lot of contact with the patient is treated differently from relatives who have little direct contact with the patient. Carers would normally be kept fully informed of the progress of the patient by the psychiatric team. A conflict of interest can develop if the patient strongly objects to the carer or relative being kept informed. Information may only be disclosed then if it has a direct effect on the health, wellbeing and safety of the carer.

The patient will usually require the carer to arrange care or help for other people who are dependent on the patient (eg, children). The patient may also wish that the carer keeps the patient's financial affairs in sufficient order so that the patient is not faced with insurmountable practical problems on discharge from hospital (eg, threat of eviction from housing because rent to the landlord has not been paid).

Relatives who provide no direct care for the patient should only be kept informed if the patient consents. The nearest relative, however, whether they have regular contact with the patient or not, has the right to appeal against detention under the 1983 Mental Health Act [10].

General practitioners

General practitioners (GPs) need to be informed of a decision to admit the patient or manage them at home for mania because they have responsibility, as the responsible medical officer (RMO), for the patient unless the patient is admitted or under the direct care of a consultant psychiatrist. Therefore, GPs have a right to know where the patient is being treated, who by and how. GPs are also an important source of information on past history and adherence to medication prescribed in primary care. They also usually provide one of the medical recommendations for detention under the 1983 Mental Health Act, as a doctor with previous knowledge of the patient.

Social workers

Approved social workers (ASWs) are qualified social workers that have passed a one-year course in the assessment of mental health problems and the interpretation of the 1983 Mental Health Act. ASWs are on duty all the time and contactable by telephone to assess patients who may be detained under the 1983 Mental Health Act [10]. Their job is to ascertain if there are any alternative treatments to compulsory hospital admission that may apply to the patient being assessed. If compulsory admission is deemed necessary, the ASW is responsible for conveying the patient to hospital, but may need the help of an ambulance, the police and sometimes the psychiatrist to do this safely. The police have to be involved if a magistrate's order is served on a patient to enter a person's home to complete a mental health assessment under the 1983 Mental Health Act, and in any situation where public order may be disrupted. It is rare for an ambulance staffed by one person to be deemed safe to transport a patient with mania to hospital.

Casualty officers and other emergency department staff

Patients with mania often present themselves, or are brought by carers or the police (section 136 of 1983 Mental Health Act), to casualty departments from the community for the purposes of psychiatric assessment. A casualty department is well-staffed, open at all times, and can rule out medical reasons for disturbed behaviour, such as head injury. Patients with mania can be disruptive, however, and casualty staff may have little specific psychiatric training. Therefore, the police should agree to stay with disruptive patients with mania. Psychiatric units should be prepared to supply nursing staff and psychiatrists at short notice to casualty departments until an assessment and appropriate disposal have been arranged under the direction of the psychiatrist.

Psychiatric hospital staff

Before a patient with mania is admitted to hospital or accepted for home treatment, it is important that the psychiatrist, who has made an assessment of the patient with mania in the community, provides information, as shown in Table 2.6, to the ward manager or team leader and hospital or team-based psychiatrist. The information is used to arrange adequate levels of staff provision and observation, medication, and a safe and secure environment to nurse the patient before the patient is transferred.

Information to be conveyed by assessing psychiatrist to ward managers, team leaders and hospital-based medical staff
Degree of restlessness, agitation, disinhibition and grandiosity
Risk to the patient or others through their behaviour, including details of recent attempts at suicide, reckless acts or violence
Psychiatric and medical comorbidity, including dehydration and nutritional state
Legal status of the patient
Immediate care plan including level of security, observation and medication
Details of carers, nearest relative and information provided to them
Action taken and required in the community to safeguard dependents and property (eg, where children have been taken)

Table 2.6

If the information is not provided, the ward manager or team leader is legally entitled to refuse to admit the patient on the grounds of safety.

Conclusion

Safe and appropriate initial management of the patient with mania in hospital or in the community requires a relevant past history and accurate clinical assessment, which identifies factors that may complicate management and risks to the patients and others. Planning, co-ordination and communication are required by the assessing psychiatrist and relatives, primary carers, frontline emergency service and specialist psychiatric staff in the hospital or community.

References

1. Altshuler LL, Post RM, Leverich GS et al. **Antidepressant-induced mania and cycle acceleration: a controversy revisited.** Am J Psychiatry 1995; **152**:1130–1138.

2. Ahlfors UG, Baastrup PC, Dencker SJ et al. **Flupenthixol decanoate in recurrent manic-depressive illness. A comparison with lithium.** Acta Psychiatr Scand 1981; **64**:226–237.

3. Swann AC, Bowden CL, Calabrese JR et al. **Mania: differential effects of previous depressive and manic episodes on response to treatment.** Acta Psychiatr Scand 2000; **101**: 444–451.

4. Tohen M, Tsuang MT, Goodwin DC. **Prediction of outcome in mania by mood-congruent or mood-incongruent psychotic features.** Am J Psychiatry 1992; **149**:1580–1584.

5. Kupfer DJ, Frank E, Grochocinski VJ et al. **Stabilization in the treatment of mania, depression and mixed states.** Acta Neuropsychiatr 2000; **12**:110–114.

6. Keller MB, Lavori PW, Coryell W et al. **Differential outcome of pure manic, mixed/cycling, and pure depressive episodes in patients with bipolar illness.** JAMA 1986; **255**:3138–3142.

7. Morriss R. **Clinical importance of inter-episode symptoms in patients with bipolar affective disorder.** J Affect Disord 2002; **72**(suppl 1):S3–S13.

8. Perry A, Tarrier N, Morriss R et al. **Randomised controlled trial of efficacy of teaching patients with bipolar disorder to identify early symptoms of relapse and obtain treatment.** BMJ 1999; **318**:149–153.

9. General Medical Council. Seeking Patient's Consent: The Ethical Considerations. London: General Medical Council; 1998.

10. Gostin L. A Practical Guide to Mental Health Law. London: MIND; 1983.

Chapter 3

Drug treatment in the initial phase of acute mania

K Macritchie, AH Young

Recent years have witnessed important advances in the understanding of bipolar disorder. With the clarification of the psychopathology found in the acute episodes of bipolar disorder and better understanding of the evolution of the underlying illness, the aims of therapeutic intervention have changed. These advances in understanding have coincided with the advent of new effective agents for the treatment of bipolar disorder. As yet, there is no perfect 'anti-manic' agent: new medications, like the old ones, have strengths and limitations. In managing mania, clinicians are now, however, better able to tailor drug treatment to the characteristics of the individual's presentation, the pattern of illness and tolerance of medication.

When defined conservatively, bipolar disorder has a lifetime incidence of 0.3–1.5 per 100. Amongst mental illnesses, bipolar disorder is one of the leading causes of worldwide disability [1]. Manic and hypomanic symptoms contribute significantly to this burden. One study examined the long-term natural history of the illness by charting the weekly symptomatic status of patients with bipolar I disorder for a mean of 12.8 years [2]. On average, bipolar I patients spent more than a year in a manic or hypomanic state. These findings highlight the need for effective and well-tolerated treatment for mania.

Assessment of a manic episode

In the management of mania, careful exploration of the symptoms of the manic episode and the underlying disease is required, as shown in Table 3.1. Awareness of the psychopathology of the manic episode, especially the presence of mixed episodes, its relationship to depressive episodes, the severity of symptoms, the presence of psychotic symptoms and cycling frequency are fundamental to successful management. Suicide risk should be assessed, especially in mixed mania. Physical aetiology should be explored. In addition, physical complications, including comorbid substance and dependence should be identified and addressed. The possibility of pregnancy in women of childbearing age should be considered. Previous response to medication, patient preference and previous experience of side effects should be ascertained.

Assessment of mania
Assessment of psychopathology of the manic episode and underlying illness
Classic versus mixed mania
Presence of psychotic symptoms
Severity of current symptoms
Suicide risk
Course of illness, especially presence of rapid-cycling disorder
Consider possibility of an organic affective disorder
Assessment of physical contributory factors
For example, endocrine disorders
Assessment of associated physical complications
Self-neglect, self-harm, dehydration or withdrawal states
Pregnancy
Previous response to medication
Identification of exacerbating agents
Presence of comorbid substance abuse or dependency
Antidepressant drugs
Steroids

Table 3.1

Pharmacological management of mania

The aim of treatment is the safe and speedy resolution of symptoms. The treatment setting and nursing measures should ensure safety and reduce over-stimulation. The basic tenets of the management of mania are:

- to achieve sedation;
- to reduce risk to self and others;
- to commence treatment with an anti-manic agent; and
- to withdraw potentially exacerbating medication, such as antidepressant agents.

The choice of anti-manic agent is partly determined by the characteristics of the manic episode and the presence of rapid-cycling disorder as detailed in Table 3.2. Other considerations include the patient's physical health and the risk of adverse effects.

Lithium

Lithium has been used in the treatment of bipolar disorder for 50 years. It has proven efficacy in the treatment of mania in classic euphoric mania, including psychotic mania, and is reported to have specific antisuicidal effects [4]. Mixed

Patterns of mania typically responding to different drug combinations			
Hypomania	**Mania**	**Mixed episode**	**Rapid-cycling disorder**
Monotherapy: lithium, valproate or an antipsychotic drug (eg, olanzapine)	Combination therapy: lithium or valproate plus an antipsychotic agent (eg, olanzapine)	Valproate If severe, add an antipsychotic agent (eg, olanzapine)	Valproate If severe, add an antipsychotic agent (eg, olanzapine) Consider benzodiazepine for agitation and insomnia
	+ consider addition of a benzodiazepine for agitation and insomnia	+ consider addition of a benzodiazepine for agitation and insomnia	Alternative agents: lithium, carbamazepine, lamotrigine
Failure of first-line medication			
Combination therapy as for severe mania	Addition of another first-line medication	Addition of another first-line medication	Combination therapy Addition of another first-line agent

Table 3.2. Notes: 1) For those who suffer recurrence while on maintenance treatment, the dose of existing medication should be optimized; 2) antidepressant drugs should be tapered and discontinued; 3) manic or mixed episodes with psychotic features usually require treatment with an antipsychotic medication; and 4) further treatment options include a change of antipsychotic drug (eg, clozapine, which may be effective in the treatment of refractory illness) or electroconvulsive therapy. Adapted with permission from American Psychiatric Association. *American Psychiatric Association Practice Guideline for the Treatment of Patients with Bipolar Disorder. Second edition.* Washington, DC: American Psychiatric Publishing; 2002 [3]. http://www.psych.org/clin_res/bipolar_revisebook_index.cfm

states and rapid-cycling disorder are, however, associated with relatively poor response rates to lithium [5,6]. The narrow therapeutic index, poor tolerability and high incidence of 'rebound mania' on withdrawal of lithium [7] further limit its effectiveness. Despite these shortcomings, lithium retains a role as a first-line treatment.

Lithium is administered orally. It equilibrates between extracellular and intracellular spaces over more than a week and a therapeutic response may be expected to begin within this time period. Therapeutic serum concentrations in mania are at the higher end of the range 0.6–1.0 mmol/l. Lithium has a heavy adverse effect burden, particularly at higher serum levels. For sedation, supplementary medication may be required initially. A benzodiazepine may be preferable to high-dose antipsychotic drugs, given the reports of encephalopathy and persistent neurological deficits that occur with the combination of lithium and haloperidol.

Anticonvulsants

The anticonvulsants, valproate and carbamazepine, are established as alternative and adjunctive treatments to lithium in bipolar disorder. Originally, anticonvulsants were used when lithium was poorly tolerated or ineffective. Now valproate is used as the first-line monotherapy for mania. The mechanism of action of anticonvulsants in bipolar disorder remains unclear.

Valproate

Valproate (2-propylpentanoic acid) is the most frequently prescribed mood stabilizer in the USA and is increasingly used in Europe. The efficacy of valproate in the treatment of mania was confirmed in a recent Cochrane Review [8]. The anti-manic efficacy of valproate, in comparison with lithium, remains uncertain. Valproate appears to be efficacious in the treatment of classic and dysphoric mania and superior to lithium in the treatment of rapid-cycling disorder, although the evidence to support this is gathered from subgroup analyses and open trials rather than controlled studies [8].

Valproate may be started at an initial dose of 750 mg, then increased by 250 mg every two-to-three days, according to response, serum levels and adverse effects. A dose of 1–3 g is usually associated with the best response. There is no clear relationship between plasma level and effect. 'Oral loading' regimens may be used to provide rapid responses in acute mania, starting at 30 mg/kg of bodyweight/day for the first two days followed by 20 mg/kg of bodyweight thereafter. The therapeutic range is 60–120 mg/l. A response may be expected in 5–10 days in the first case and in three days for 'oral loading'.

Valproate is available in several forms, including sodium valproate, valproic acid and depakote (divalproex or valproate semi-sodium), a compound of sodium valproate and valproic acid. Both sodium valproate and valproate semi-sodium are effective in the treatment of acute mania [9–11]. There are no trials directly comparing the efficacy of available forms. Methodologically rigorous studies comparing the pharmacokinetics, efficacy and tolerability of valproate and divalproex are required.

Carbamazepine

Carbamazepine is reported to be effective in randomized controlled trials in mania, although methodological difficulties, such as small numbers and adjunctive medication, limit the evidence base for its use. One placebo-controlled crossover study in which no adjunctive medication was used, found that 63% of carbamazepine-treated patients displayed significant improvement in manic, depressive and psychotic symptoms; an effect that was lost on switching to placebo [12]. Lithium was superior to carbamazepine in one randomized controlled trial [13], while another reported them to be of equal efficacy [14]. Valproate was found to be superior to carbamazepine in a randomized controlled trial [15]. Open trials suggest a role for carbamazepine in rapid-cycling and mixed state disorders [16]. Carbamazepine may be started at 200 mg twice daily, aiming for a serum therapeutic range of 6–12 mg/l. Response may be expected in 14 days.

New anticonvulsants

Recently, the role of other anticonvulsants, such as lamotrigine, gabapentin and topiramate, has been investigated. An initial small controlled trial suggested some efficacy for lamotrigine in mania, but the evidence for its efficacy in bipolar depression and rapid-cycling disorder is stronger [17–20]. The use of gabapentin in mania, suggested by open trials is not supported by randomized controlled data [20]. Preliminary open observations of adjunctive topiramate treatment suggest that it may have anti-manic or anti-cycling effects in bipolar disorder [21]. Oxcarbamazepine, a keto-analogue of carbamazepine with less induction of 3A4 enzymes, has been reported to have anti-manic effects, but more methodologically robust data are awaited.

Typical antipsychotic drugs

Typical antipsychotic drugs are effective in acute mania, but may exacerbate post-manic depression. Their onset of action is possibly faster than that of lithium, although lithium may exert superior efficacy with regard to affective symptoms in milder states. Some antipsychotic drugs (eg, chlorpromazine) may be more effective in addressing psychomotor agitation [22].

Antipsychotic medication may be started at doses equivalent to chlorpromazine 75–300 mg or haloperidol 3 mg three times daily. When indicated, zuclopenthixol acetate may be administered with an initial dose of 50–150 mg, repeated after two-to-three days with a maximum cumulative dose of 400 mg over two weeks. Depot typical antipsychotic drugs (eg, flupenthixol decanoate or flupenthazine decanoate) may be useful. In all cases, caution is required when typical antipsychotic drugs are co-administered with lithium.

Atypical antipsychotic drugs

Of the atypical antipsychotic drugs, olanzapine has the largest evidence base in bipolar disorder. It has been shown to be superior to valproate in the treatment of mania [23] and in 2000, it was approved by the Food and Drug Administration (FDA) for the short-term treatment of acute manic episodes associated with bipolar I disorder. Olanzapine is efficacious in the treatment of both psychotic and non-psychotic mania [24]. Open trials and case reports also support the use of olanzapine in mixed states. The use of risperidone in mania is supported by a large open trial [25] and controlled data is anticipated shortly. Olanzapine may be started at 10 mg/day, risperidone at 2 mg twice daily. Rapid-release forms of olanzapine and risperidone are now available.

There is increasing evidence that ziprasidone and quetiapine also have anti-manic effects. The prototype atypical antipsychotic drug, clozapine, is frequently reserved for use in highly refractory cases of bipolar disorder. No double-blind, controlled studies of clozapine in the treatment of acute bipolar mania have been published, but several open reports support the anti-manic and antipsychotic efficacy of clozapine in bipolar disorder, including classic (pure) and mixed mania and rapid-cycling disorder.

Combination treatments for mania

The use of combination treatments is increasingly common, but little evidence yet exists. The anti-manic effects of lithium in combination with carbamazepine [26,27] have been the studied in controlled trials, which suggest synergistic action. Several studies have supported the use of add-on atypical antipsychotic drugs, including risperidone, to improve outcomes in bipolar disorder [28]. A recent study supported the use of olanzapine with valproate or lithium for the treatment of mania in patients partially non-responsive to valproate or lithium monotherapy [29].

Treatment strategies

An outline of treatment strategies is shown in Table 3.2. Clearly, a history of good response to an anti-manic agent should help inform the first choice of treatment. Otherwise, lithium or valproate should be used in classic mania; valproate should be prescribed for dysphoric mania or rapid-cycling disorder. Of the newer agents, olanzapine is a potential first-line treatment. If the first choice is only partially successful, then a second anti-manic agent should be added. If mania persists, then a combination of three agents should be used, possibly with the addition of an atypical antipsychotic drug.

In practice, initial sedation is usually required, particularly if there is marked psychomotor agitation or insomnia. Often sedative and mood stabilizing medication are commenced together. If psychotic symptoms are present or symptoms are severe, then use of an antipsychotic medication is preferred. Otherwise, a benzodiazepine may be used. Benzodiazepines are useful adjunctive sedative or hypnotic agents. Both lorazepam and clonazepam have demonstrated efficacy in the treatment of mania. For example, a randomized, double-blind clinical study examined haloperidol in comparison to lorazepam as adjunctive treatment to lithium for mania [30]. There was no significant difference between the two treatment groups in the magnitude of, or time to, response. Antipsychotic drugs and benzodiazepines may be used in combination.

The use of short-term medications should be reviewed regularly and the doses of benzodiazepine and/or antipsychotic drug adjusted according to response. These medications should be discontinued when symptoms resolve; withdrawal after a 12-week period is common.

Non-pharmacological treatment

A review of English language reports of the use of electroconvulsive therapy (ECT) in mania concluded that it was an efficacious treatment for mania [31]. It was associated with remission or marked clinical improvement in 80% of patients with mania and appeared to be an effective treatment for patients whose manic episodes responded poorly to pharmacotherapy. The authors were, however, unable to draw conclusions regarding the issue of relapse following ECT, its effects on cognition and the benefits of unilateral ECT in comparison to bilateral ECT in patients with mania. Analysis of therapeutic trials conducted over a 16-year period suggest that ECT followed by lithium maintenance is superior in efficacy to treatment with lithium or antipsychotic drugs in hospitalized patients with mania [32].

New non-pharmacological treatments, such as transcranial magnetic stimulation (TMS) and vagal nerve stimulation, are emerging. The evidence for TMS in the treatment of mania remains small. One controlled trial of repetitive TMS in mania demonstrated that stimulation of the right prefrontal cortex produced a greater improvement in mania than left hemisphere stimulation [33]. This study was, however, methodologically weakened by the absence of a sham-treated control group. There are also reports of TMS-induced hypomania [34].

Psychological treatment

Psychological treatments, such as cognitive behavioural therapy, may be used to target recognition of early warning symptoms. This technique depends on the maintenance of insight. One study demonstrated that teaching patients to recognise early symptoms of manic relapse and to seek early treatment was associated with improvements in the time to first manic relapse [35].

Conclusion

Manic symptoms contribute substantially to the burden of disease in bipolar disorder. Recently, the pharmacological management of manic episodes has been greatly strengthened by the introduction of several new anti-manic agents, notably valproate and several atypical antipsychotic drugs, especially olanzapine. Although the evidence base for these agents is growing, more methodologically rigorous studies are required, particularly in the area of combination treatment.

The treatment of mania should not be considered in isolation. The choice of medication should be undertaken following consideration of the context of the underlying bipolar illness and the necessity for continuation and maintenance phases of treatment. Psychological and nursing measures should complement pharmacological intervention.

In the future, as the understanding of mania and bipolar disorder agents develops, so the concept of therapeutic targets will evolve and new anti-manic agents will emerge. The progress of recent years may offer encouragement to clinicians and patients as they attempt to understand and manage this complex and fascinating disorder.

References

1. Murray CJ, Lopez AD. **Global mortality, disability, and the contribution of risk factors: Global Burden of Disease Study.** *Lancet* 1997; **349**:1436–1442.

2. Judd LL, Akiskal HS, Schettler PJ *et al*. **The long-term natural history of the weekly symptomatic status of bipolar I disorder.** *Arch Gen Psychiatry* 2002; **59**:530–537.

3. American Psychiatric Association. *American Psychiatric Association Practice Guideline for the Treatment of Patients with Bipolar Disorder. Second edition.* Washington, DC: American Psychiatric Publishing; 2002.

4. Thies-Flechtner K, Muller-Oerlinghausen B, Seibert W *et al*. **Effect of prophylactic treatment on suicide risk in patients with major affective disorders. Data from a randomized prospective trial.** *Pharmacopsychiatry* 1996; **29**:103–107.

5. Swann AC, Bowden CL, Calabrese JR *et al*. **Pattern of response to divalproex, lithium, or placebo in four naturalistic subtypes of mania.** *Neuropsychopharmacology* 2002; **26**:530–536.

6. Dunner DL, Patrick V, Fieve RR. **Rapid cycling manic depressive patients.** *Compr Psychiatry* 1977; **18**:561–566.

7. Goodwin GM. **Recurrence of mania after lithium withdrawal. Implications for the use of lithium in the treatment of bipolar affective disorder.** *Br J Psychiatry* 1994; **164**:149–152.

8. Macritchie KAN, Geddes JR, Scott J *et al*. **Valproate for acute mood episodes in bipolar disorder.** *Cochrane Database Syst Rev* 2003; **1**:CD004052 .

9. Freeman TW, Clothier JL, Pazzaglia P *et al*. **A double-blind comparison of valproate and lithium in the treatment of acute mania.** *Am J Psychiatry* 1992; **149**:108–111.

10. Pope HG Jr, McElroy SL, Keck PE Jr *et al*. **Valproate in the treatment of acute mania. A placebo-controlled study.** *Arch Gen Psychiatry* 1991; **48**:62–68.

11. Bowden CL, Brugger AM, Swann AC *et al*. **Efficacy of divalproex vs lithium and placebo in the treatment of mania. The Depakote Mania Study Group.** *JAMA* 1994; **271**:918–924.

12. Ballenger JC, Post RM. **Therapeutic effects of carbamazepine in affective illness: a preliminary report.** *Commun Psychopharmacol* 1978; **2**:159–175.

13. Lerer B, Moore N, Meyendorff E *et al*. **Carbamazepine versus lithium in mania: a double-blind study.** *J Clin Psychiatry* 1987; **48**:89–93.

14. Small JG, Klapper MH, Milstein V *et al*. **Carbamazepine compared with lithium in the treatment of mania.** *Arch Gen Psychiatry* 1991; **48**:915–921.

15. Vasudev K, Goswami U, Kohli K. **Carbamazepine and valproate monotherapy: feasibility, relative safety, and efficacy and therapeutic drug monitoring in manic disorder.** *Psychopharmacology* 2000; **150**:15–23.

16. Post RM, Uhde TW, Roy-Byrne PP *et al*. **Correlates of antimanic response to carbamazepine.** *Psychiatry Res* 1987; **21**:71–83.

17. Ichim L, Berk M, Brook S. **Lamotrigine compared with lithium in mania: a double-blind randomized controlled trial.** *Ann Clin Psychiatry* 2000; **12**:5–10.

18. Calabrese JR, Suppes T, Bowden CL *et al*. **A double-blind, placebo-controlled, prophylaxis study of lamotrigine in rapid-cycling bipolar disorder. Lamictal 614 Study Group.** *J Clin Psychiatry* 2000; **61**:841–850.

19. Calabrese JR, Bowden CL, Sachs GS *et al*. **A double-blind placebo-controlled study of lamotrigine monotherapy in outpatients with bipolar I depression. Lamictal 602 Study Group.** *J Clin Psychiatry* 1999; **60**:79–88.

20. Frye MA, Ketter TA, Kimbrell TA *et al*. **A placebo-controlled study of lamotrigine and gabapentin monotherapy in refractory mood disorders.** *J Clin Psychopharmacol* 2000; **20**:607–614.

21. Grunze HC, Normann C, Langosch J *et al*. **Antimanic efficacy of topiramate in 11 patients in an open trial with an on-off-on design.** *J Clin Psychiatry* 2001; **62**:464–468.

22. Prien RF, Caffey EM Jr, Klett CJ. **Comparison of lithium carbonate and chlorpromazine in the treatment of mania. Report of the Veterans Administration and National Institute of Mental Health Collaborative Study Group.** *Arch Gen Psychiatry* 1972; **26**:146–153.

23. Tohen M, Jacobs TG, Grundy SL *et al*. **Efficacy of olanzapine in acute bipolar mania: a double-blind, placebo-controlled study. The Olanzapine HGGW Study Group.** *Arch Gen Psychiatry* 2000; **57**:841–849.

24. Tohen M, Baker RW, Altshuler LL *et al*. **Olanzapine versus divalproex in the treatment of acute mania.** *Am J Psychiatry* 2002; **159**:1011–1117.

25. Vieta E, Herraiz M, Parramon G *et al*. **Risperidone in the treatment of mania: efficacy and safety results from a large, multicentre, open study in Spain.** *J Affect Disord* 2002; **72**:15–19.

26. Small JG, Klapper MH, Marhenke JD *et al*. **Lithium combined with carbamazepine or haloperidol in the treatment of mania.** *Psychopharmacol Bull* 1995; **31**:265–272.

27. Kramlinger KG, Post RM. **Adding lithium carbonate to carbamazepine: antimanic efficacy in treatment-resistant mania.** *Acta Psychiatr Scand* 1989; **79**:378–385.

28. Miller DS, Yatham LN, Lam RW. **Comparative efficacy of typical and atypical antipsychotics as add-on therapy to mood stabilizers in the treatment of acute mania.** *J Clin Psychiatry* 2001; **62**:975–980.

29. Tohen M, Chengappa KN, Suppes T *et al*. **Efficacy of olanzapine in combination with valproate or lithium in the treatment of mania in patients partially nonresponsive to valproate or lithium monotherapy.** *Arch Gen Psychiatry* 2002; **59**:62–69.

30. Lenox RH, Newhouse PA, Creelman WL *et al*. **Adjunctive treatment of manic agitation with lorazepam versus haloperidol: a double-blind study.** *J Clin Psychiatry* 1992 **53**:47–52.

31. Mukherjee S, Sackeim HA, Schnurr DB. **Electroconvulsive therapy of acute manic episodes: a review of 50 years' experience.** *Am J Psychiatry* 1994; **151**:169–176.

32. Small JG, Klapper MH, Milstein V *et al*. **Comparison of therapeutic modalities for mania.** *Psychopharmacol Bull* 1996; **32**:623–627.

33. Grisaru N, Chudakov B, Yaroslavsky Y *et al*. **Transcranial magnetic stimulation in mania: a controlled study.** *Am J Psychiatry* 1998; **155**:1608–1610.

34. Garcia-Toro M. **Acute manic symptomatology during repetitive transcranial magnetic stimulation in a patient with bipolar depression.** *Br J Psychiatry* 1999; **175**:491.

35. Perry A, Tarrier N, Morriss R *et al*. **Randomised controlled trial of efficacy of teaching patients with bipolar disorder to identify early symptoms of relapse and obtain treatment.** *BMJ* 1999; **318**:149–153.

Chapter 4

Follow-up of patients recovering from the acute phase

ML Phillips, MJ Travis

The interventions for the maintenance and follow-up of bipolar patients recovering from acute episodes of mania are briefly outlined in this chapter. In particular, the importance of compliance with medication in patients with bipolar disorder, the structuring of outpatient follow-up and the management of drug therapy in the intermediate phase of treatment are discussed.

Compliance with medication

In over 90% of bipolar patients, functional recovery often lags behind symptomatic and syndromal recovery, with recurrent episodes appearing to lead to progressive deterioration in recovery, and the number of episodes potentially affecting subsequent treatment response and prognosis [1–4]. It has been shown that, of patients hospitalized during a manic or mixed episode of bipolar illness, only 26% have symptomatic recovery, and only 24% functional recovery after one year [5]. Similar low rates for functional recovery have been found after two years [6]. In addition to the low functional recovery, relapse is common. In the first year after an index episode up to 50% of patients will have either a manic or depressive relapse, rising up to 75% after four years [2,7].

A major problem in patients with mood disorders is the high level of noncompliance with medication [8,9]. This has been associated with increased rates of admission to psychiatric hospitals [9,10] and a lower level of syndromic recovery in patients hospitalized for a manic or mixed episode of illness after one year [5]. Poor compliance with medication in patients with mood disorders may be related to attitudes about psychotropic medication [9] and poor insight into the nature of psychiatric illness [11], particularly during manic episodes and in patients with psychotic symptoms [12,13]. In patients recovering from a manic or mixed episode of illness, poor compliance with medication has also been associated with comorbid substance abuse [14]. Comorbid substance abuse is particularly associated with patients with a history of mania [15]. Although this association may be showed by patients who have had manic episodes as a result of substance misuse, other studies have indicated that comorbid substance abuse may have a lifetime prevalence of up to 61% in patients with bipolar I disorder [16]. It occurs in 42% of outpatients with bipolar disorder of any kind [17].

Despite this, few studies have examined the extent to which altering attitudes towards medication and insight about psychiatric illness can affect compliance with medication in patients with mania. In comparison, studies of patients with schizophrenia have demonstrated that improving attitudes towards medication and insight about psychiatric illness and symptoms can increase compliance with medication [18,19].

Follow-up

Major priorities for the management of patients recovering from an acute manic episode are:

- encouragement of compliance with medication;
- increasing awareness and detection of early signs of relapse of illness;
- management of lifestyle to avoid risk of illness relapse; and
- organization of long-term outpatient psychiatric care for the management of symptoms of the disorder and comorbid conditions, including substance abuse [20].

Improving compliance with medication

There is increasing evidence demonstrating that compliance with medication in patients with bipolar disorder often fails within the first few months of treatment [21]. In bipolar patients, encouraging the belief that medication can be helpful in treating psychiatric illness, increasing motivation for medication use [22] and the establishment of a regular habit for taking medication can help to increase compliance with medication [20]. Simplification of medication regimens, so that patients are prescribed fewer rather than larger numbers of different mood stabilizers and/or antipsychotic medications, and involvement of social support systems (including family and/or friends), may also encourage patients to comply with medication regimens.

Awareness and early detection of signs of relapse of illness

Awareness and early detection of signs of relapse of illness are clearly important in the long-term management of bipolar disorder, although it is important to distinguish early symptoms of manic relapse from residual symptoms of the last bipolar relapse and other causes of symptoms, such as comorbidity with other psychiatric disorders. Early detection of signs of relapse and appropriate intervention strategies by patients and support systems have been demonstrated to reduce significantly the number of manic episodes [23]. Early detection and intervention have been emphasised in cognitive-behavioural strategies for the treatment of bipolar disorder [24,25].

Management of lifestyle and stress

Lifestyle management includes the protection of the sleep–wake cycle, together with structuring of daily schedules to allow a balance between activity and relaxation [19]. The onset of mania has been associated with a significantly greater number of disruptions in the sleep–wake cycle than the onset of depression in bipolar patients [26]. These disruptions can include shift work, crossing time zones or even early morning appointments. It is important to note that sleep loss in particular has been associated with the development of mania [27]. The engagement of social support systems to help patients minimize the occurrence of factors leading to lifestyle disruption and increases in stress has been emphasised, therefore, as an important component of the management of bipolar disorder [28].

Structuring outpatient management

It is crucially important that patients are provided with adequate outpatient psychiatric care. Ideally, care should be co-ordinated by a specific member of the community mental health team, with provision of a community psychiatric nurse, to ensure regular monitoring of mental state, medication compliance and social support, and management of psychiatric illness and comorbid anxiety and substance abuse. In a recent report, it has been suggested that regular contact with patients by telephone on some occasions may also be helpful in assessing certain, but not all, clinical features of bipolar illness [29]. Access to emergency support facilities outside normal hours and regular communication with primary care teams ensure that additional support systems are available to the patient and can help provide the main care co-ordinator with further information regarding the patient's mental health and medication compliance. Referral for cognitive behaviour therapy, family therapy or specialist services, as appropriate, should be considered if the patients have beliefs that are unhelpful in managing their bipolar disorder (eg, 'There is nothing that I can do to prevent mania'), there is friction and hostility to the patient or the patient does not adequately respond to first or second-line treatments for maintenance of bipolar disorder.

Managing drug therapy

Prevention of a relapse into mania

It is apparent that manic episodes recur in roughly 90% of patients with bipolar affective disorder over their lifetimes. A significant proportion of these relapses occur during the first 12 months after initial diagnosis and may relate to noncompliance with treatment and the well-established link between sudden cessation of mood stabilizers (especially lithium) and abrupt relapse [30]. Furthermore, up to 70% of patients recovering from an episode of mania still suffer from residual affective symptoms [31], which could potentially interfere with service engagement and increase the risk of early relapse.

One of the primary aims during this phase of treatment is the optimization of pharmacological therapies as a prelude to the long-term treatment and prophylaxis of bipolar affective disorder. With regard to mood stabilizers, there is increasing evidence that these should be started as early in the course of bipolar affective disorder as possible [32]. This is considered in further detail in the next chapter.

There are, however, some important issues that need to be addressed in this intermediate phase of treatment.

Benzodiazepines

During the acute phase of mania it is common (and recommended in most guidelines) to add a benzodiazepine to whatever medication is used as the primary therapy in mania. Once the manic symptoms have begun to subside the benzodiazepine must be withdrawn to prevent over-sedation and subsequent dependence.

The recommended reduction schedule is to reduce the total dose of benzodiazepine by a quarter every week to two weeks depending on clinical state. Faster reductions can be considered if the patient is over-sedated or has only been on benzodiazepines for a few days [33].

If the patient is receiving a shorter-acting benzodiazepine, such as lorazepam or clonazepam, it may be prudent to switch them to a longer-acting benzodiazepine, such as diazepam, as this decreases the risk of the withdrawal phenomena.

Antipsychotic drugs

In the UK, antipsychotic drugs are the first-line treatment for an acute manic episode, particularly if the episode is associated with psychotic symptoms. On the available evidence this probably represents good practice. Up to two-thirds of patients will still be receiving antipsychotic drugs six months to two years after their index manic episode [3,34]. Previously because of extrapyramidal adverse effects seen with the older typical antipsychotic drugs there was an impetus and need to reduce and stop these medications as soon as practicable after manic symptom resolution. This was in order to prevent long-term adverse effects, especially as these seem to be more prevalent in bipolar patients taking antipsychotic drugs than in patients with schizophrenia [35]. Nevertheless the older typical antipsychotic drugs did appear to confer benefits in terms of relapse prevention into mania in bipolar affective disorder, but may have increased the risk of depression [36].

The more recently introduced 'atypical' antipsychotic drugs do not appear to cause neurological adverse effects to the same extent as the older typical antipsychotic drugs. Although there are increasing concerns over some of their long-term metabolic effects, in the medium term phase of treatment considered here there is little need to consider a reduction or cessation of 'atypical' antipsychotic treatment that has been effective in the acute phase. In the longer term, maintenance phase of bipolar affective disorder there is increasing evidence to recommend the use of some of the newer medications, particularly olanzapine [37].

Prevention of future depression

In the medium-term phase of treatment, it is often important to consider the previous manic episodes that a patient may have suffered. If these were invariably followed by a depressive episode the clinician may wish to consider offering the patient prophylaxis for the risk of developing depression.

There is a consensus that the best medications for the prophylaxis of depressive episodes in bipolar affective disorder are mood-stabilizers given alone [38], with a suggestion that the mood stabilizer of choice would be lamotrigine. This remains to be fully tested.

There is little evidence to confirm a suitable strategy for antidepressant drug use in these cases. Most studies with newer antidepressant drugs have been initiated after the onset of depressive symptoms. Considering the available evidence, there would be little to recommend the use of tricyclic antidepressant drugs in these circumstances as there is reasonable data which suggest an association between this class of medication and a switch back into mania [39]. This risk appears to be present, but much reduced, in patients treated with selective serotonin reuptake inhibitors (SSRIs), therefore their use may be safer. The use of SSRIs in conjunction with mood-stabilizers is recommended in established severe cases of depression in bipolar affective disorder.

Rapid-cycling bipolar disorder

This is a feature of bipolar affective disorder that may only become apparent after an acute manic episode when the patient's mood cycle begins to rapidly oscillate between mania/hypomania and depression. This change in the character of illness may be induced by antidepressant drugs [38]. Other causes to exclude are biochemical hypothyroidism (sometimes lithium induced) and comorbid substance misuse. Generally, antidepressant drugs should be stopped and lithium therapy reduced and stopped in these patients. The limited evidence available suggests that valproate and carbamazepine are the treatments of choice [40] and there is also recent increasing evidence for lamotrigine.

Conclusions

The management of bipolar patients recovering from acute mania during the intermediate phase of treatment has been discussed. The complex nature of bipolar disorder and the specific issues to be addressed in the psychosocial and pharmacological management of these patients has been emphasised.

In the longer term, decisions will need to be made by the multi-disciplinary team regarding the level of involvement of primary, secondary and tertiary services to optimize treatment on an individual basis, whilst aiming to improve patient insight and compliance with medication. It is important to remember to involve the patient and support systems in all levels of this decision making process.

References

1. Dion GL, Tohen M, Anthony WA et al. **Symptoms and functioning of patients with bipolar disorder six months after hospitalization.** *Hosp Community Psychiatry* 1998; **39**:652–657.

2. Tohen M, Waternaux CM, Tsuang MT. **Outcome in mania. A 4-year prospective follow-up of 75 patients utilizing survival analysis.** *Arch Gen Psychiatry* 1990; **47**:1106–1111.

3. Keck PE Jr, McElroy SL, Strakowski SM. **Anticonvulsants and antipsychotics in the treatment of bipolar disorder.** *J Clin Psychiatry* 1998; **59**(suppl 6):74–81.

4. Keck PE Jr, McElroy SL, Strakowski SM et al. **12-month outcome of patients with bipolar disorder following hospitalization for a manic or mixed episode.** *Am J Psychiatry* 1998; **155**:646–652.

5. Tohen M, Hennen J, Zarate CM Jr et al. **Two-year syndromal and functional recovery in 219 cases of first-episode major affective disorder with psychotic features.** *Am J Psychiatry* 2000; **157**:220–228.

6. Goldberg JF, Harrow M, Grossman LS. **Course and outcome in bipolar affective disorder: a longitudinal follow-up study.** *Am J Psychiatry* 1995; **152**:379–384.

7. Gitlin MJ, Swendsen J, Heller TL et al. **Relapse and impairment in bipolar disorder.** *Am J Psychiatry* 1995; **152**:1635–1640.

8. Jamison KR, Gerner RH, Goodwin FK. **Patient and physician attitudes toward lithium: relationship to compliance.** *Arch Gen Psychiatry* 1979; **36**:866–869.

9. Pope M, Scott J. **Do clinicians understand why individuals stop taking lithium?** *J Affect Disord* 2003; **74**:287–291.

10. Colom F, Vieta E, Martinez-Aran A et al. **Clinical factors associated with treatment noncompliance in euthymic bipolar patients.** *J Clin Psychiatry* 2000; **61**:549–555.

11. Ghaemi SN, Pope HG Jr. **Lack of insight in psychotic and affective disorders: a review of empirical studies.** *Harv Rev Psychiatry* 1994; **2**:22–33.

12. Peralta V, Cuesta MJ. **Lack of insight in mood disorders.** *J Affect Disord* 1998; **49**:55–58.

13. Yen CF, Chen CS, Yeh ML et al. **Comparison of insight in patients with schizophrenia and bipolar disorder in remission.** *J Nerv Ment Dis* 2002; **190**:847–849.

14. Keck PE Jr, McElroy SL, Strakowski SM et al. **Compliance with maintenance treatment in bipolar disorder.** *Psychopharmacol Bull* 1997; **33**:87–91.

15. Kessler RC, Nelson CB, McGonagle KA et al. **The epidemiology of co-occurring addictive and mental disorders: implications for prevention and service utilization.** *Am J Orthopsychiatry* 1996; **66**:17–31.

16. Regier DA, Farmer ME, Rae DS et al. **Comorbidity of mental disorders with alcohol and other drug abuse. Results from the Epidemiologic Catchment Area (ECA) Study.** *JAMA* 1990; **264**:2511–2518.

17. McElroy SL, Altshuler LL, Suppes T et al. **Axis I psychiatric comorbidity and its relationship to historical illness variables in 288 patients with bipolar disorder.** *Am J Psychiatry* 2001; **158**:420–426.

18. Kemp R, Kirov G, Everitt B et al. **Randomised controlled trial of compliance therapy. 18-month follow-up.** *Br J Psychiatry* 1998; **172**:413–419.

19. Healey A, Knapp M, Astin J *et al.* **Cost-effectiveness evaluation of compliance therapy for people with psychosis.** *Br J Psychiatry* 1998; **172**:420–424.

20. Otto MW, Reilly-Harrington N, Sachs GS. **Psychoeducational and cognitive-behavioural strategies in the management of bipolar disorder.** *J Affect Disord* 2003; **73**:171–181.

21. Johnson RE, McFarland BH. **Lithium use and discontinuation in a health maintenance organization.** *Am J Psychiatry* 1996; **153**:993–1000.

22. Rollnick S, Miller WR. **What is motivational interviewing?** *Behav Cogn Psychother* 1995; **23**:334.

23. Perry A, Tarrier N, Morriss R *et al.* **Randomised controlled trial of efficacy of teaching patients with bipolar disorder to identify early symptoms of relapse and obtain treatment.** *BMJ* 1999; **318**:149–153.

24. Lam DH, Watkins ER, Hayward P *et al.* **A randomized controlled study of cognitive therapy for relapse prevention for bipolar affective disorder: outcome of the first year.** *Arch Gen Psychiatry* 2003; **60**:145–152.

25. Newman CF, Leahy RL, Beck AT *et al.* *Bipolar Disorder: A Cognitive Therapy Approach.* Washington, DC: American Psychiatric Association; 2001.

26. Malkoff-Schwartz S, Frank E, Anderson B *et al.* **Stressful life events and social rhythm disruption in the onset of manic and depressive bipolar episodes: a preliminary investigation.** *Arch Gen Psychiatry* 1998; **55**:702–707.

27. Wehr TA. **Sleep-loss as a possible mediator of diverse causes of mania.** *Br J Psychiatry* 1991; **159**:576–578.

28. Scott J. **Cognitive therapy for clients with bipolar disorder.** *Cogn Behav Pract* 1996; **3**:19–51.

29. Brar LK, Brar JS, Deily NG *et al.* **Can clinical features of bipolar-1 disorder be assessed reliably on the telephone?** *J Affect Disord* 2002; **71**:221–227.

30. Baldessarini RJ, Tondo L, Faedda GL *et al.* **Effects of the rate of discontinuing lithium maintenance treatment in bipolar disorders.** *J Clin Psychiatry* 1996; **57**:441–448.

31. Gitlin MJ, Swendsen J, Heller TL *et al.* **Relapse and impairment in bipolar disorder.** *Am J Psychiatry* 1995; **152**:1635–1640.

32. Goldberg JF, Ernst CL. **Features associated with the delayed initiation of mood stabilizers at illness onset in bipolar disorder.** *J Clin Psychiatry* 2002; **63**:985–991.

33. Taylor D, McConnell H, Duncan-McConnell D *et al.* *The South London and Maudsley NHS Trust 2001 Prescribing Guidelines. 6th edition.* London: Martin Dunitz; 2001.

34. Verdoux H, Gonzales B, Takei N *et al.* **A survey of prescribing practice of antipsychotic maintenance treatment for manic-depressive outpatients.** *J Affect Disord* 1996; **38**:81–87.

35. Kusumakar V. **Antidepressants and antipsychotics in the long-term treatment of bipolar disorder.** *J Clin Psychiatry* 2002; **63**(suppl 10):23–28.

36. Ahlfors UG, Baastrup PC, Dencker SJ *et al.* **Flupenthixol decanoate in recurrent manic-depressive illness. A comparison with lithium.** *Acta Psychiatr Scand* 1981; **64**:226–237.

37. Yatham LN. **The role of novel antipsychotics in bipolar disorders.** *J Clin Psychiatry* 2002; **63**(suppl 3):10–14.

38. Sachs GS, Printz DJ, Kahn DA *et al.* **The expert consensus guideline series: medication treatment of bipolar disorder 2000.** *Postgrad Med* 2000; Special Report:1–104.

39. Altshuler LL, Post RM, Leverich GS *et al.* **Antidepressant-induced mania and cycle acceleration: a controversy revisited.** *Am J Psychiatry* 1995; **152**:1130–1138.

40. Calabrese JR, Fatemi SH, Kujawa M *et al.* **Predictors of response to mood stabilizers.** *J Clin Psychopharmacol* 1996; **16**(suppl 1):24S–31S.

Chapter 5

Long-term follow-up of mania

JC Cookson

Natural history and prognosis of bipolar disorder

The great majority of patients with mania have more than one episode because bipolar disorder is a recurrent illness. The onset may become more rapid in later episodes. The average interval from one episode to the next tends to decrease during the first five episodes, for example, from five years between the first and second episode to two years between the fifth and sixth [1–3], as shown in Figure 5.1. In an individual there is, however, great variability in the length between episodes and a tendency for clustering at times of particular stress. Relapses tend to cluster together followed by a quiescent period followed by relapses clustering together over the patient's life. A long interval between the first and second episode is especially likely if the first episode followed adverse life events. There is an increased rate of life events in the month before mania, but the proportion of patients affected is small and the first episode is more likely to be triggered by life events than later episodes. This is in keeping with the suggestion that a process of 'kindling' occurs facilitating the development of subsequent episodes. Insomnia or sleep deprivation may trigger a manic episode, for example, when flying overnight from west to east or in parents following childbirth.

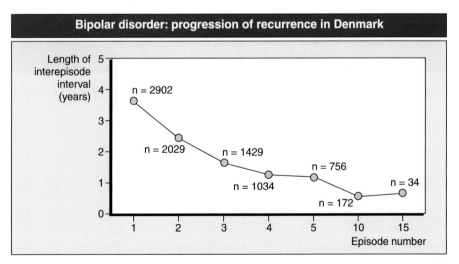

Figure 5.1. Adapted with permission from Kessing LV, Andersen PK, Mortensen PB *et al*. **Recurrence in affective disorder. I. Case register study.** *Br J Psychiatry* 1998; **72**:23–28 [2].

Patients may increase or decrease alcohol or drug abuse when manic or depressed. Alcohol or abuse of stimulant drugs can alter the course of bipolar disorder by triggering mania; they diminish impulse control, impair judgement and are serious risk factors for suicide. Cannabis may increase psychotic symptoms in mania and induce mania, as may cocaine and other psychostimulants. Therefore, the recognition and treatment of alcohol and drug abuse in bipolar patients is a matter of urgency.

Outcome

Before effective treatment was available, approximately 20% of hospitalized patients with mania died, many from exhaustion. With modern treatment, increased mortality from natural causes occurs only in those with a concurrent physical illness. Later death by suicide, however, occurs in approximately 15–20% of cases [4]. A proportion of patients become socially and economically disadvantaged. There can be a considerable social and economic burden on the family. Table 5.1 shows the outcomes in a follow-up in Boston of 166 people with first episode mania [5]. It should be noted that approximately 50% of people in this group had mood-incongruent psychotic features, associated with a poorer prognosis.

Prophylaxis of bipolar disorder

Selection of patients

Maintenance treatment should always be considered after a second episode of bipolar disorder, especially if the interval between episodes was less than five years [6,7].

Recovery and new illness episodes within two years of a first-lifetime hospitalization for mania	
Event	**Number (%)**
Index episode	166 (100)
Syndromally recovered	155 (93.4)
Functionally recovered	58 (34.9)
New episode	65 (41.9)
Relapse	2 (1.3)
Recurrence	55 (35.5)
Switch	8 (5.2)
None	90 (58.1)
New episode type	
Mania	33 (21.3)
Depression	32 (20.7)

Table 5.1. Data from Tohen M, Hennen J, Zarate CM Jr *et al.* **Two-year syndromal and functional recovery in 219 cases of first-episode major affective disorder with psychotic features.** *Am J Psychiatry* 2000; **157**:220–228. **[5].**

Because the intervals between the first and second episodes tend to be longer than between subsequent episodes, maintenance treatment should only be used after a first episode if the dangers of a subsequent episode are thought to justify it; for example, if the episode was severe and disruptive, had a relatively sudden onset and was not precipitated by external factors or if the person's job is very sensitive or there is a risk of suicide.

Lithium maintenance

Patients who are more likely to benefit from lithium are those with typical bipolar disorder having complete recovery between episodes, or a family history of bipolar disorder. Patients with a rapid-cycling phase of illness are less responsive to lithium [8]. Other factors militating against prophylactic efficacy are poor adherence to treatment and drug abuse.

Importance of adherence to treatment

A large proportion of patients at risk do not seek treatment and many who do nonetheless adhere poorly to lithium. There is also the risk of withdrawal mania in those who stop treatment too abruptly, for example, when feeling no need for it during a mild upswing of mood. Because of this risk, prolonged lithium treatment should not be proposed in patients who are likely to comply poorly [9]. Where steps are taken to encourage and check adherence, however, low relapse rates and affective morbidity on lithium can be achieved. This is part of the rationale for specialist lithium or affective disorder clinics or for shared care protocols.

Patients are less likely to adhere if they are younger, male and have had fewer previous episodes. The reasons they give for stopping are its ineffectiveness, drug adverse effects, feeling well and in no need of treatment, finding it inconvenient and not wanting to depend on medication and feeling less energy or drive. The adverse effects most often given as reasons are:

- excessive thirst and polyuria;
- tremor;
- memory impairment; and
- weight gain [10].

Improving adherence and outcome

In order to increase adherence, the doctor should take adverse effects seriously, keep lithium levels as low as possible, educate the patients and their families about the illness and the use of lithium and discuss adherence with the patient. Pharmacists should be able to provide information sheets about lithium for the patient and cards on which doctors can record blood test results and doses. Sometimes manipulation of dose schedules can be helpful, for example, switching from once to twice daily doses or if patients have individual preferences. Regular contact and counselling can be useful. It may be helpful to plot a 'life chart' with the patient, to improve their understanding of the impact of their condition. It may also be helpful to give them a daily 'mood chart' or 'diary' to complete and bring for review at their next appointment, particularly if their mood has been unstable.

In spite of these measures many bipolar patients tend to drop out of lithium treatment. Cognitive therapy may be helpful by altering the patients understanding and attitude towards their illness and treatment and, therefore, improving compliance. Some patients do not adhere to lithium because of lack of effectiveness; these patients may benefit from an increase in the dose of lithium within therapeutic limits because higher doses of lithium reduce affective morbidity (relapses and inter-episode symptoms), but also increase adverse effects and possibility of toxicity [11,12].

Lithium lessens both the severity and the frequency of episodes. Usually it also stabilizes the mood between major episodes. A five-year follow-up conducted in Naples of all patients commenced on lithium, showed only 23% continuing on it without recurrence for five years, as shown in Table 5.2 [13]. Another 29% had continued lithium and suffered a recurrence, but had a reduction in the amount of hospitalization by more than 50% compared with the pretreatment period. Only 39% of the patients were managed for five years on lithium alone. Most of those who stopped lithium did so on their own initiative; the most common reasons given were:

- perceived ineffectiveness (37%);
- adverse effects (28%);
- no need for the medication (18%);
- found it inconvenient (12%); or
- felt a loss of drive (5%) [13].

Long-term outcome of lithium prophylaxis	
Patients still on lithium	61%
With no recurrence of episodes	23%
With some recurrence, but with >50% decrease in hospitalization	29%
At end point	
Patients on lithium alone	39%
Patients on no psychotic drugs except benzodiazepines	6%

Table 5.2. Reproduced with permission from Maj M, Pirozzi R, Magliano L *et al.* **Long-term outcome of lithium prophylaxis in bipolar disorder: a 5-year prospective study of 402 patients at a lithium clinic.** *Am J Psychiatry* 1998; **155**:30–35 [13].

The mortality rate (high because of suicides and cardiovascular deaths) can be reduced on lithium [10].

Clinical trials: the evidence

The methodology for demonstrating the efficacy of a drug, such as lithium, in long-term prophylaxis is the prospective, parallel group, double-blind, placebo-controlled trial with random allocation.

Placebo-controlled studies of lithium prophylaxis

Two large prospective randomized placebo-controlled trials and five smaller studies have been reported. Overall, in 204 patients on lithium prospectively, approximately 35% relapsed in the study period (which varied from four months to three years), compared with approximately 80% of 221 patients on placebo [1]. In 1973, the study of Prien *et al.* [14] was particularly positive and is summarized in Table 5.3 using the number needed to treat format.

Relapse and dropout rates and NNT in a two-year lithium trial of patients with bipolar disorder		
	Lithium (n = 101)	Placebo (n = 104)
Dropout due to lack of efficacy (%)	11	40
Dropout due to adverse events (%)	1	0
Relapse (%)	43	81
Absolute risk reduction (%)	38	
NNT (95% CI)	3 (3–4)	

Table 5.3. NNT, number needed to treat; CI, confidence interval. Adapted with permission from Cookson JC, Katona C, Taylor D. *Use of Drugs in Psychiatry: The Evidence from Psychopharmacology. Fifth edition.* London: The Royal College of Psychiatrists/Gaskell; 2002 [15].

The efficacy of lithium was more apparent for manic than for depressive relapses. Lithium improves both the severity and frequency of episodes. It also usually stabilizes the mood between major episodes. The reduction in depression may be secondary to the prevention of mania, which would otherwise be followed by a post-manic depressive phase.

Blood levels and monitoring

Blood levels of lithium lower than those for acute mania are sufficient in prophylaxis (0.5–1.0 mmol/l). For some patients lower levels than this would suffice. In the elderly a level of 0.5 mmol/l is recommended. During less stable phases lithium levels should be undertaken frequently and even in the most stable the tests of lithium level, renal and thyroid function should be performed at least once a year.

Antidepressant drugs and lithium

Lithium reduces the risk of switching into mania during treatment with anti-depressant drugs. Depression occurring during lithium treatment can be treated with monoamine reuptake inhibitors. Most psychiatrists would recommend selective serotonin reuptake inhibitors (SSRIs) rather than tricyclic anti-depressant drugs or monoamine oxidase inhibitors (MAOIs) initially because of the risk of interactions with other drugs and foods (with MAOIs) and because SSRIs have lower switch rates than either tricyclic antidepressant drugs or MAOIs. In patients with bipolar I disorder the course of antidepressant treatment should be gradually discontinued as the depression improves, in order to reduce the risk of triggering a manic episode and to avoid the induction of rapid cycling. For patients with a predominantly depressive pattern of disorder (including bipolar II disorder), long-term treatment with lithium is more effective than imipramine or placebo, but the combination of lithium and a monoamine reuptake inhibitor may be more effective in preventing depression than either drug alone. SSRIs, such as paroxetine, are less liable to induce mania than the tricyclic antidepressant drugs. Some bipolar patients are, however, readily switched into mania on particular SSRIs.

Discontinuation of lithium

In bipolar patients abrupt cessation of lithium leads to the development of mania two-to-three weeks later in up to 50%. This should be part of the information given to patients starting on lithium. Discontinuation should be gradual, certainly over more than two weeks and preferably at the rate of one quarter to one eighth of the original dose every two months. Patients whose mood has been stable are less likely to relapse on stopping than those who have continued to show mild mood swings ('metastable'). Discontinuation over four weeks appears to carry a much lower risk of early recurrence than abrupt discontinuation.

Lithium toxicity

Clinical features

Lithium can produce many adverse effects, but toxicity is indicated by the development of three groups of symptoms:

- gastrointestinal;
- motor (especially cerebellar);
- and cerebral, as shown in Table 5.4.

Diagnosis of toxicity

Lithium toxicity should be assumed in patients on lithium with vomiting or severe nausea, cerebellar signs or disorientation. Lithium treatment should be stopped

Symptoms resulting from lithium toxicity			
	Gastrointestinal	**Motor/cerebellar**	**Cerebral**
Mild	Nausea Diarrhoea	Severe fine tremor	Poor concentration
Moderate	Vomiting	Coarse tremor Cerebellar ataxia Slurred speech	Drowsiness Disorientation
Severe	Vomiting Incontinence	Choreiform/Parkinsonian movement General muscle twitching (myoclonus) Spasticity and cerebellar dysfunction EEG abnormalities and seizures	Apathy Coma

Table 5.4. EEG, electroencephalograph. Adapted with permission from Cookson JC, Katona C, Taylor D. *Use of Drugs in Psychiatry: The Evidence from Psychopharmacology. Fifth edition.* London: The Royal College of Psychiatrists/Gaskell; 2002 [15].

immediately and serum lithium, urea and electrolyte levels measured. The severity of toxicity bears little relationship to serum lithium levels, however, and neurotoxicity can occur with serum levels in the usual therapeutic range. Diagnosis should be based on clinical judgement and not on the blood level. Lithium should only be re-started (at an adjusted dose) when the patient's condition has improved or an alternative cause of the symptoms has been found.

Outcome

Patients who survive episodes of lithium toxicity will often make a full recovery, but some have persistent renal or neurological damage with cerebellar symptoms, spasticity and cognitive impairment. This outcome is more likely if patients are continued on lithium while showing signs of toxicity.

Factors predisposing to lithium toxicity

Conditions of salt depletion (diarrhoea, vomiting, excessive sweating during fever or in hot climates) can lead to lithium retention. Drugs that reduce the renal excretion of lithium include: thiazide diuretics (but not frusemide or amiloride), certain non-steroidal anti-inflammatory drugs (indometacin, piroxicam, naproxen and phenylbutazone, but not aspirin, paracetamol or sulindac), certain antibiotics (erythromycin, metronidazole and probably tetracyclines) and calcium antagonists. If these drugs are used, the dose of lithium should be reduced and blood levels monitored.

In patients with serious intercurrent illnesses, especially infections, lithium should be stopped or reduced in dose and carefully monitored until the patient's condition is stable. Gastroenteritis is particularly likely to lead to toxicity. In the elderly, renal function is decreased, lower doses are required and toxicity can develop more readily.

Alternatives to lithium in long-term treatment

Even in favourable clinical trials lithium maintenance is unsuccessful in over 30% of patients and more recent studies, which include a broader range of patients with mania, put the failure rate much higher. Coupled with the problems of discontinuation mania and the risk of neurotoxicity, there is clearly a need for alternative drugs.

Carbamazepine

For lithium non-responders an alternative is carbamazepine. Patients with rapid-cycling are more likely to benefit from carbamazepine than from lithium. In longer-term use, there may be partial loss of efficacy by the third year, although it is not clear to what extent poor adherence to medication is responsible. Two recent trials have shown, however, a substantial advantage to lithium compared with carbamazepine in preventing relapse [16].

Adverse effects of carbamazepine can be minimized by using slow-release formulations or by commencing treatment with low doses (100–200 mg at night) and increasing every few days to the maximum dose that is well tolerated (usually 400–600 mg, maximum 1600 mg/day). Patients should be informed of the risk of adverse effects, including blood disorders, and told to report possible symptoms, such as sore throat, rash or fever, to the doctor.

Valproate

Valproate (as divalproex) has been studied in one placebo-controlled, double-blind, randomized trial [17], which showed rates for all relapses of 24% in the valproate-treated patients compared with 38% in placebo-treated patients. For the primary outcome measure, survival time to a new manic or depressive episode, there was no significant difference between divalproex or lithium compared with placebo. A high proportion of patients in the study were previously regarded as non-responders to lithium. Divalproex was superior to placebo in terms of lower rates of discontinuation for either a recurrent mood episode or depressive episode. In fact the effect on depressive relapse was higher than that on manic relapse in this study.

Lamotrigine

Two large clinical trials have compared lamotrigine, lithium and placebo [18,19]. In one the index episode was mania and in the other depression. Both trials showed a significant advantage for lamotrigine over lithium in the prophylaxis of depression. There was a comparable advantage for lithium over lamotrigine for mania, but the effects of lamotrigine against depression were relatively slight and not clearly different from lithium. For lithium and lamotrigine, there was a trend to prevent both poles of the illness.

Thus, the strongest evidence in prophylaxis is still for lithium. Lamotrigine may help in predominantly depressed bipolar patients such as those with bipolar

II disorder including rapid-cycling bipolar II [20] and bipolar I patients following a depressive episode.

Long-term treatment with antipsychotic drugs

Antipsychotic drugs should be avoided, if possible, for long-term use in bipolar patients because of sedative effects and, in the case of typical antipsychotics, tardive dyskinesia. Brief intermittent therapy is possible in which the patient commences an antipsychotic drug, particularly at night, when they sense a period of lability of mood, racing thoughts or insomnia. For those who have frequently recurring episodes and either do not benefit from, or do not adhere to, oral medication, depot antipsychotic medication can, however, provide long periods of stability [21].

Olanzapine plus lithium or valproate has been shown to be more effective than lithium or valproate alone for preventing mania during the subsequent 12 months in a placebo-controlled relapse prevention study in bipolar I patients whose recent manic episode had settled on a combination of lithium or valproate plus olanzapine [22].

Thus, atypical antipsychotics, such as olanzapine, may prove to have a greater role in the long-term follow-up of patients after a manic episode than the typical antipsychotics.

Combination treatments

For long-term treatment of bipolar disorder monotherapy is not usually sufficient and it attracts polypharmacy, which may be necessary, but can lead to the creation of a 'drug fog'. In such cases, if possible, medication should be limited to mood-stabilizing drugs and an antipsychotic drug or an antidepressant drug. Daily mood charting is helpful to document changes associated with the introduction or removal of individual drugs. Some patients benefit more from the combination of lithium and carbamazepine than from either drug alone, but reversible neurological adverse effects can occur, characterized mainly by confusional states and cerebellar signs similar to those of lithium toxicity. The combination of lithium with valproate produces less neurological problems [23]. Carbamazepine is difficult to combine with drugs other than lithium because it is a potent inducer of liver enzymes that can then metabolize the drugs.

Conclusion

Recurrent affective disorder carries a poor prognosis in terms of frequency of episodes, divorce, physical illness and suicide. Bipolar affective disorder is also compatible with periods of successful leadership, productivity and creativity. Treatment can reduce the disruption of personal function and may reduce the mortality and suicide risk. Sufferers from this condition should be educated concerning the nature of their condition and the treatments available and should be encouraged to choose effective treatment and to use it to best advantage.

References

1. Goodwin FK, Jamison KR. *Manic-Depressive Illness.* Oxford: Oxford University Press; 1990.

2. Kessing LV, Andersen PK, Mortensen PB *et al.* **Recurrence in affective disorder. I. Case register study.** *Br J Psychiatry* 1998; **172**:23–28.

3. Marneros A, Angst J. *Bipolar Disorders: 100 Years after Manic-depressive Insanity.* Dordrecht: Kluwer Academic Publishers; 2000.

4. Muller-Oerlinghausen B, Berghofer A. **Antidepressants and suicidal risk.** *J Clin Psychiatry* 1999; **60**(suppl 2):94–99.

5. Tohen M, Hennen J, Zarate CM Jr *et al.* **Two-year syndromal and functional recovery in 219 cases of first-episode major affective disorder with psychotic features.** *Am J Psychiatry* 2000; **157**:220–228.

6. American Psychiatric Association. *American Psychiatric Association Practice Guidelines for the Treatment of Patients with Bipolar Disorder. 2nd edition.* Washington, DC: American Psychiatric Association; 2002.

7. Frances AJ, Kahn DA, Carpenter D *et al.* **The expert consensus guidelines for treating depression in bipolar disorder.** *J Clin Psychiatry* 1998; **59**(suppl 4):73–79.

8. Wehr TA, Sack DA, Rosenthal NE *et al.* **Rapid cycling affective disorder: contributing factors and treatment responses in 51 patients.** *Am J Psychiatry* 1988; **145**:179–184.

9. Cookson J. **Lithium: balancing risks and benefits.** *Br J Psychiatry* 1997; **171**:120–124.

10. Cookson JC, Sachs GS. **Lithium: clinical use in mania and prophylaxis of affective disorders.** In: *Schizophrenia and Mood Disorders: The New Drug Therapies in Clinical Practice.* Edited by PF Buckley and JL Waddington. Oxford: Butterworth Heinemann, 1999;155–178.

11. Gelenberg AJ, Kane JM, Keller MB *et al.* **Comparison of standard and low serum levels of lithium for maintenance treatment of bipolar disorder.** *N Engl J Med* 1989; **321**:1489–1493.

12. Keller MB, Lavori PW, Kane JM *et al.* **Subsyndromal symptoms in bipolar disorder. A comparison of standard and low serum levels of lithium.** *Arch Gen Psychiatry* 1992; **49**:371–376.

13. Maj M, Pirozzi R, Magliano L *et al.* **Long-term outcome of lithium prophylaxis in bipolar disorder: a 5-year prospective study of 402 patients at a lithium clinic.** *Am J Psychiatry* 1998; **155**:30–35.

14. Prien RF, Caffey EM Jr, Klett CJ. **Prophylactic efficacy of lithium carbonate in manic-depressive illness. Report of the Veterans Administration and National Institute of Mental Health collaborative study group.** *Arch Gen Psychiatry* 1973; **28**:337–341.

15. Cookson JC, Katona C, Taylor D. *Use of Drugs in Psychiatry: The Evidence from Psychopharmacology. Fifth edition.* London: The Royal College of Psychiatrists/Gaskell; 2002.

16. Greil W, Kleindienst N, Erazo N *et al.* **Differential response to lithium and carbamazepine in the prophylaxis of bipolar disorder.** *J Clin Psychopharmacol* 1998; **18**:455–460.

17. Bowden CL, Calabrese JR, McElroy SL *et al.* **A randomized, placebo-controlled 12-month trial of divalproex and lithium in treatment of outpatients with bipolar I disorder. Divalproex Maintenance Study Group.** *Arch Gen Psychiatry* 2000; **57**:481–489.

18. Bowden CL, Calabrese JR, Sachs G *et al.* **A placebo-controlled 18-month trial of lamotrigine and lithium maintenance treatment in recently manic or hypomanic patients with bipolar I disorder.** *Arch Gen Psychiatry* 2003; **60**:392–400.

19. Calabrese JR, Shelton MD, Rapport DJ *et al.* **Bipolar disorders and the effectiveness of novel anticonvulsants.** *J Clin Psychiatry* 2002; **63**(suppl 3):5–9.

20. Calabrese JR, Suppes T, Bowden CL *et al.* **A double-blind, placebo-controlled, prophylaxis study of lamotrigine in rapid-cycling bipolar disorder. Lamictal 614 Study Group.** *J Clin Psychiatry* 2000; **61**:841–850.

21. Cookson JC. **Use of antipsychotic drugs and lithium in mania.** *Br J Psychiatry* 2001; **178**(suppl 41):48–56.

22. Tohen M, Chengappa KNR, Suppes T *et al.* **Efficacy of olanzapine in combination with valproate or lithium in the treatment of mania in patients partially nonresponsive to valproate or lithium monotherapy** *Arch Gen Psychiatry* 2002; **59**:62–69.

23. Freeman MP, Stoll AL. **Mood stabilizer combinations: a review of safety and efficacy.** *Am J Psychiatry* 1998; **155**:12–21.

Appendix

Manic Depression Fellowship
21 St George's Road, London, SE1 6ES.
Telephone: 020 7793 2600.

For information, a newsletter and local support groups.

Website: www.mdf.org.uk

Index